Department of Theatre & Dance
Mary Washington College

BEHIND THE SCENES WITH AMERICA'S HOTTEST MEN

Michael Ives
Jim Palmer
Rick Edwards
Jeff Aquilon
Tom Hintnaus
Andy Warhol
Thom Fleming
Todd Irvin
Scott Webster
Marcus Abel
Attila Von Somogyi
Andrew Smith
Sinjin Smith
Buzzy Kerbox
Ron Greschner
Rich Wiese
Jason Savas
Bill Curry
Michael Holder
Charles Williamson

They're the ones who catch our eyes in magazines, on billboards, and on fashion runways. Earning an average of $125,000 a year, they're more than just tall, dark, and handsome – these men are America's fantasies come true. And now, through intimate, candid portraits in words and photos, we can finally meet the real guys behind the slick looks, the men of our dreams who have made it to the top because they're –

NOT JUST ANOTHER PRETTY FACE

NOT JUST ANOTHER PRETTY FACE

AN INTIMATE LOOK AT AMERICA'S TOP MALE MODELS

by Karen Hardy

Profiles written by Josh Reid
Design by Robert J. Luzzi

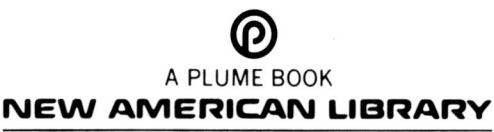

A PLUME BOOK
NEW AMERICAN LIBRARY
TIMES MIRROR
NEW YORK AND SCARBOROUGH, ONTARIO

NAL BOOKS ARE AVAILABLE AT QUANTITY DISCOUNTS WHEN USED TO PROMOTE PRODUCTS OR SERVICES. FOR INFORMATION PLEASE WRITE TO PREMIUM MARKETING DIVISION, THE NEW AMERICAN LIBRARY, INC., 1633 BROADWAY, NEW YORK, NEW YORK 10019.

Copyright © 1983 by Karen Hardy

All rights reserved.

Original photographs for this book taken by Karen Hardy

PLUME TRADEMARK REG. U.S. PAT. OFF. AND FOREIGN COUNTRIES
REGISTERED TRADEMARK—MARCA REGISTRADA
HECHO EN CRAWFORDSVILLE, IND., U.S.A.

SIGNET, SIGNET CLASSICS, MENTOR, PLUME, MERIDIAN and NAL BOOKS
are published *in the United States* by The New American Library, Inc.,
1633 Broadway, New York, New York 10019,
in Canada by The New American Library of Canada Limited,
81 Mack Avenue, Scarborough, Ontario M1L 1M8

Library of Congress Cataloging in Publication Data
Hardy, Karen.
   Not just another pretty face.

   1. Photography of men. 2. Men—Portraits. 3. Models,
Fashion—Portraits. I. Title.
TR681.M4H37   1983   799'.23   82-22540
ISBN 0-452-25395-0 (pbk.)

First Printing, April, 1983

1 2 3 4 5 6 7 8 9

PRINTED IN THE UNITED STATES OF AMERICA

**Dedicated To
The Men In This Book**

CONTENTS

Preface	ix
Rick Edwards	11
Michael Ives	17
Jim Palmer	23
Attila Von Somogyi	29
Charles Williamson	35
Jeff Aquilon	41
Tom Hintnaus	47
Buzzy Kerbox	53
Marcus Abel	59
Andrew Smith	64
Sinjin Smith	65
Ron Greschner	77
Jason Savas	83
Todd Irvin	89
Scott Webster	95
Andy Warhol	101
Rich Wiese	105
Bill Curry	111
Michael Holder	117
Thom Fleming	123
Acknowledgments	128

Preface

What are these men really like?

That was a question I heard over and over again from friends intrigued by my photography and, I suspect, my subject matter. Men have always fascinated me. Perhaps, ultimately, this is the reason I came to do this book.

The men profiled in this book are more than just successful models. Their personalities are diverse. They come from Greenfield, Massachusetts, and Kailua, Hawaii; they are business tycoons and award-winning athletes. These men entered the modeling profession in various ways—through the suggestion of a friend or solicitation by a fashion photographer, art director, or agent. Some started modeling in college, others to earn an extra buck on the side. What keeps them in it is the money. The men in this book travel to exotic locations, receive tremendous public exposure that can help them in other careers, and earn between $40,000 and $200,000 a year. They see modeling as a means to give them the freedom to pursue their other interests.

With their rugged, all-American good looks, these men exemplify a new awareness that being in shape and looking good are important—at work as well as in the bedroom. People stand in awe of these men because they've seen them on TV commercials or in *Gentleman's Quarterly (GQ), Vogue,* and other magazine spreads. Often the men in this book are insecure about being valued for the looks and not for themselves. Todd Irvin labeled it "the dilemma of the good-looking man." These men are not one-dimensional, and it is revealing to see the human side behind the flawless image.

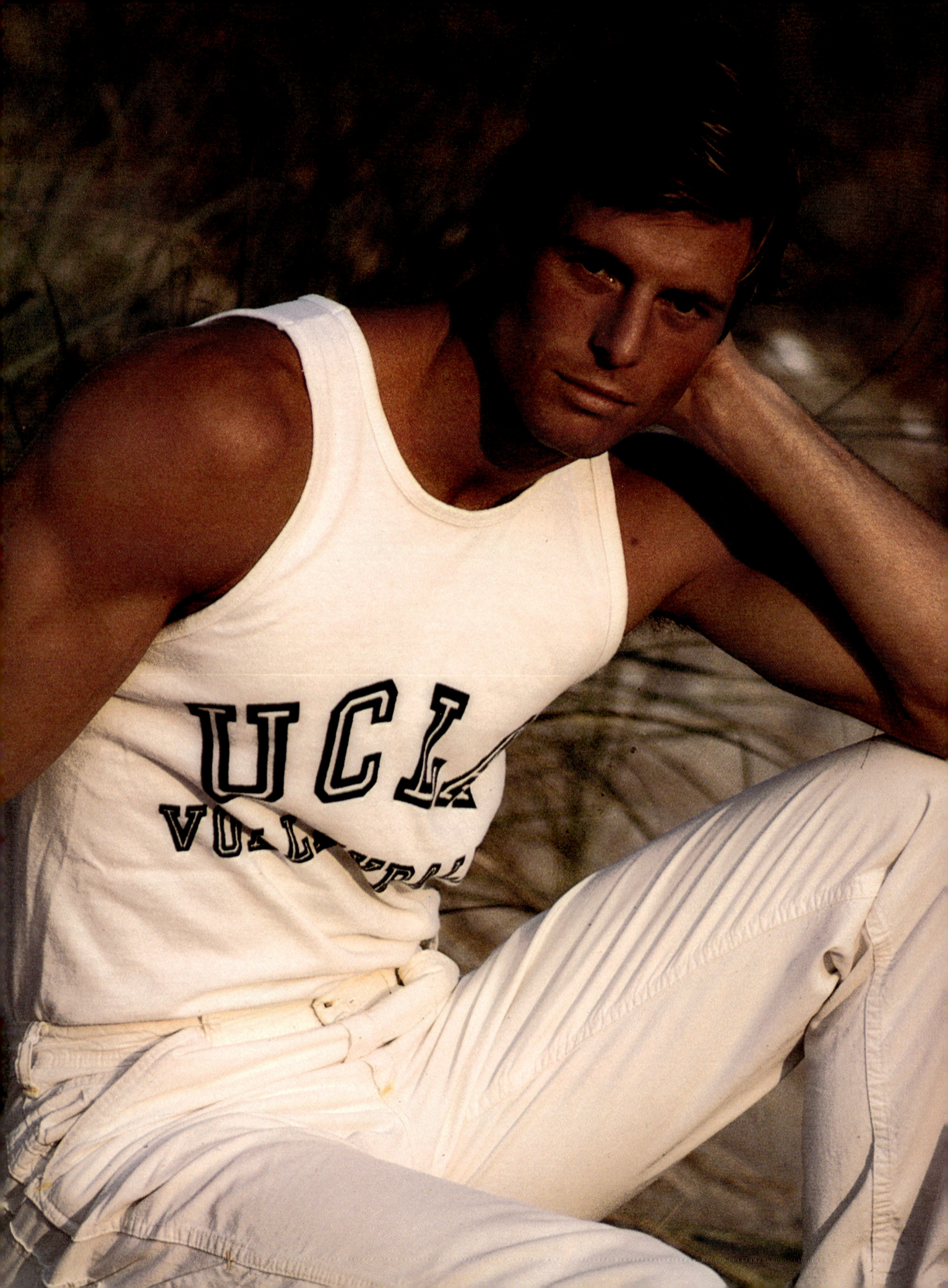

Rick Edwards

Rick Edwards is always going places: Portofino, Italy, for a fashion shoot; coast to coast on his Honda 450; to Sicily for a film; or onto a New York river for a rigorous crew workout. "When I'm not doing something, I go crazy," says Rick, who always seems to be doing *some* thing. "I don't let a minute go by if I can use it. If I've got thirty minutes before I have to go out to dinner, I'll do a workout, thirty minutes of nonstop calisthenics."

Sandy-haired and strapping, Rick Edwards may look like a California cowboy, but, at heart, he's a pure-bred East Coast Yankee. Rick learned his deeply ingrained work ethic the old-fashioned way: as a youngster helping out on the farms in Northfield, Massachusetts, the small town where he grew up. And Rick still adheres to the Yankee values that prevailed there. "In that town," he recalls, "what people did was *work*. My dad was tough, a hard-ass who believed in working twelve hours a day. I've always wanted to be busy — to prove myself to my parents and myself."

A square-jawed athlete with a friendly, lopsided grin, Rick gets immense satisfaction out of physical exertion. He held a range of strenuous jobs before gravitating toward modeling: Rick labored in a lumber mill, loaded trucks in a warehouse, and cleaned the stables at a girls' school. Although he enjoyed the physical activity, he didn't feel that his life then had much focus. "Just kicking around was terrible," Rick says. "I like hard work, but it's very frustrating when it doesn't lead anywhere. After two years, I realized I just couldn't live like that anymore."

As he pursued a degree in exercise science, Rick demanded tough physical challenges in athletics as well. During senior year at college, he won weight-lifting championships even though he was competing against guys thirty pounds heavier than himself. "I got in great shape," he says, "because I wanted more than anything else to be

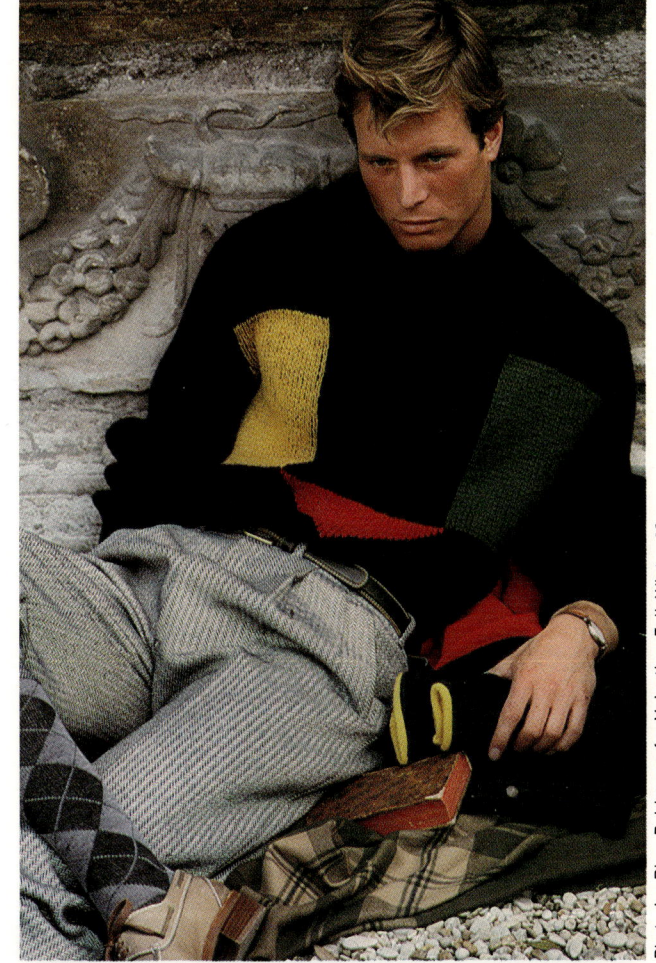

Photo by Rico Puhlmann for Valentino Fall–Winter 82

Valentino UOMO

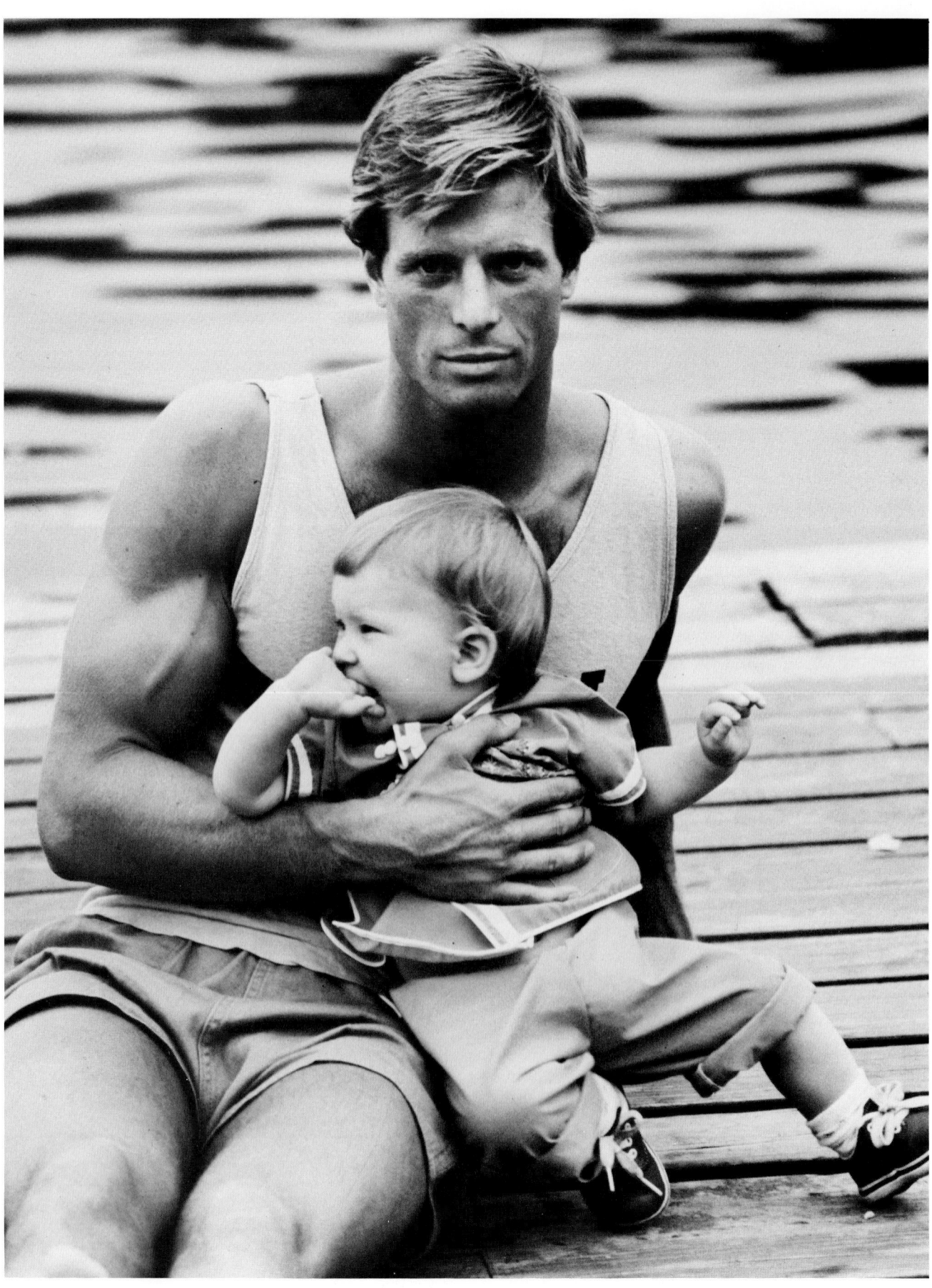

With his daughter, Jacqueline.

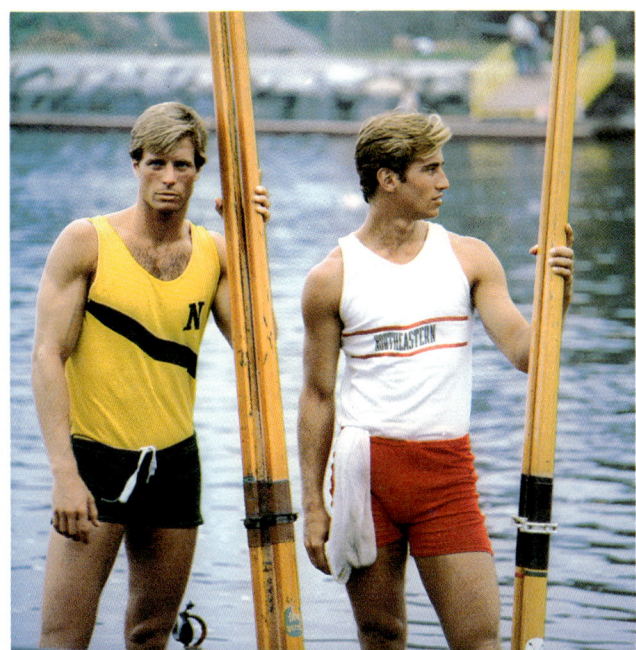

*Rick with Michael Ives at the Rowing Club:
"It's so beautiful rowing on the water. I just forget everything. It's total concentration on the boat. I row in a single shell now, a lot of times at night. It's beautiful, especially when it's quiet and the stars are out."*

able to beat everybody." Rick was also a championship rower, who trained for eight hours a day.

After graduation from college, Rick asked his coach where the best crew club was. As Rick recalls, "He said the New York Athletic Club. So I trained at the Athletic Club all summer long to make a world team." With the Athletic Club crew, Rick won the first-place trophy in the prestigious American Nationals Race and went to the World Championship in Copenhagen. Rowing led indirectly to his modeling career. On the way back from Copenhagen, Rick met an actress-model in an airport, and she suggested that he consider work in television commercials. After meeting her manager, Rick embarked on a professional career — with some misgivings. "I really didn't think I could carry it off," he says. "I didn't think I was as good-looking as some of those people." Tuxedoed and dapper, Rick appeared on the December 1981 cover of *GQ,* and has been much in demand ever since. That suits Rick fine: being on the go is what he wants to be.

To satiate his desire for perpetual motion, Rick owns not one but two Austin-Healey convertibles, and he looks forward to racing some day. "I really need that incredible, on-the-edge, near-death kind of excitement. It really tears me apart inside, but I just love it. And I'm so high when I get it." During his cross-country motorcycle trip a few years ago, Rick tempted fate with daredevil stunts.

"I'd get a little bored on the bike," he recalls. "So almost every day, I stood up on the seat of the motorcycle — for laughs. I'd get it going sixty miles an hour, then I'd stand up on the seat — one foot a little ahead of the other. I'd let go of the handlebars and just cruise down the highway. I was always searching for a thrill. I always needed that adrenaline."

Rick, who favors jeans and denim shirts that match his Pacific-blue eyes, maintains his taut frame with a regimen of rowing, running, weight lifting, and calisthenics. Now separated from his wife, Rick spends as much time as possible with his young daughter, Jacqueline. "She steals my heart," says Rick. Always pushing himself to the limit, Rick is juggling two careers: modeling and acting. His feature-film debut is the lead role in *Hearts in Armor,* a Crusades romance in which Rick is ideally cast as the shining white knight who rides to the rescue. "Where I'm going now is movies," says Rick. But what he wants out of movies — and everything else — is a certifiable challenge. "I don't mind working hard," says Rick, "but I don't want to be bored. I feel like I have all this energy and I want to *accomplish* things."

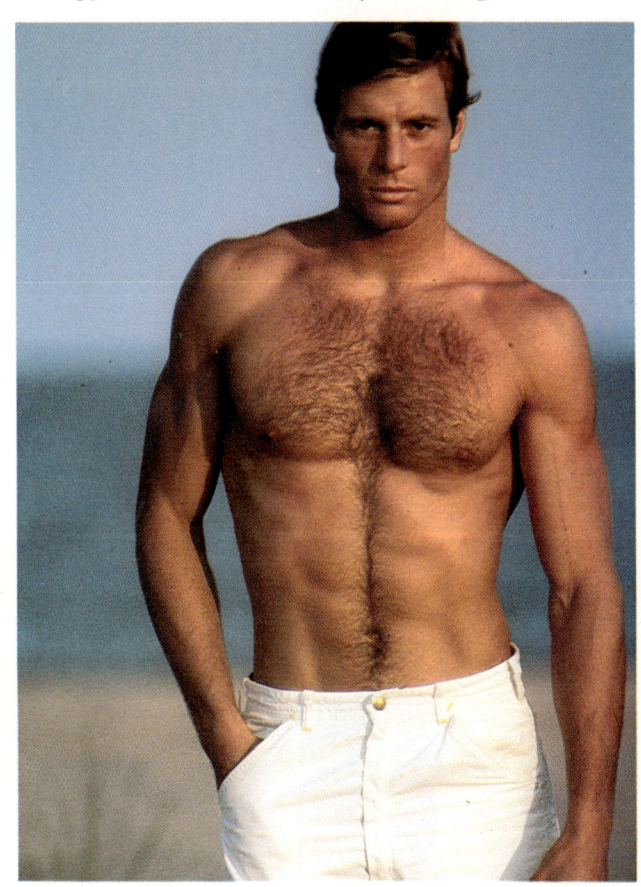

13

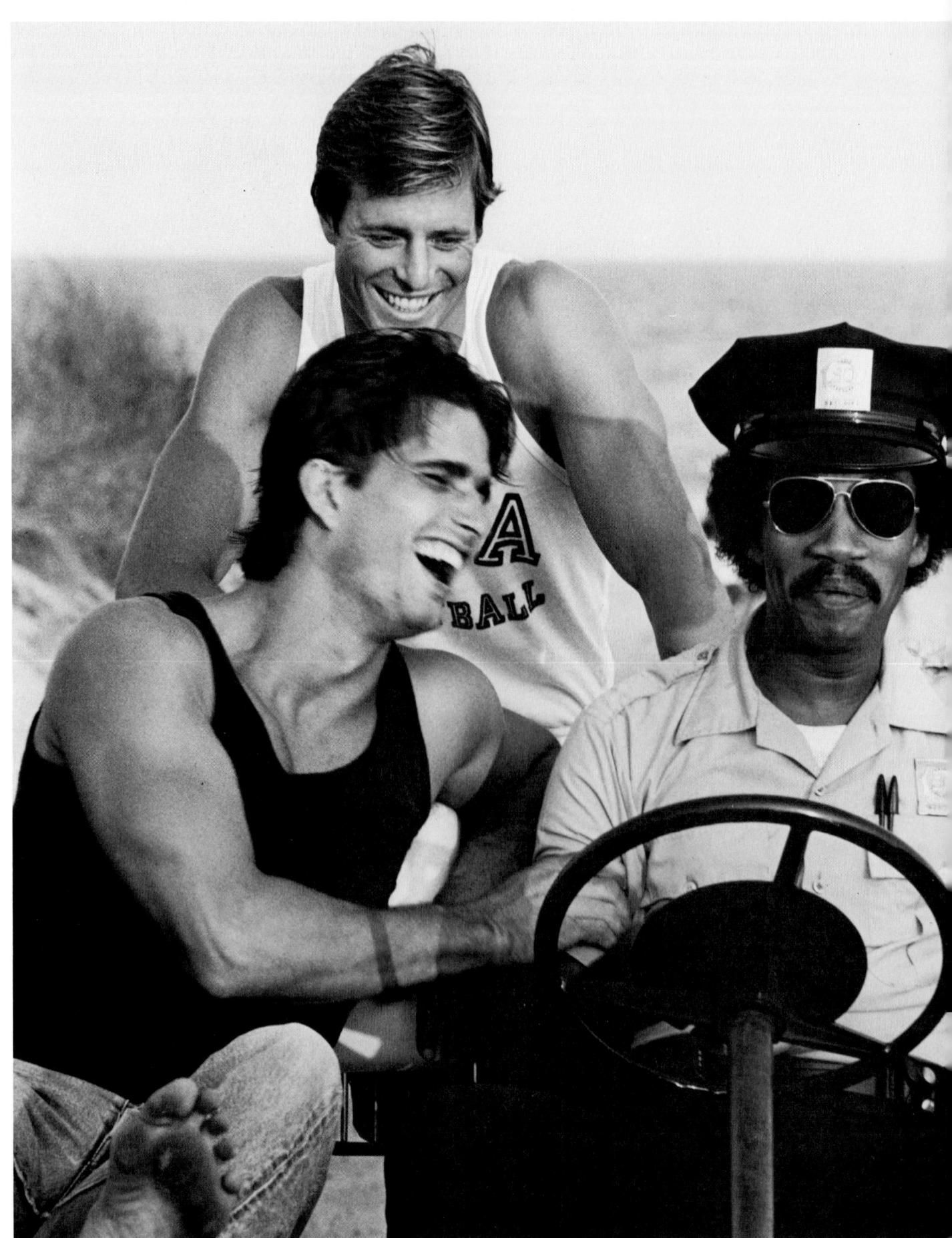

Rick with Thom Fleming and Skip in Southampton, New York.

"
I'm not the kind of person
that goes out after work
and has a couple of drinks
with someone.
I'm kind of selfish with my time.
I work, then I work out
usually. No one can really
follow me.
I'm alone and busy every minute.
"

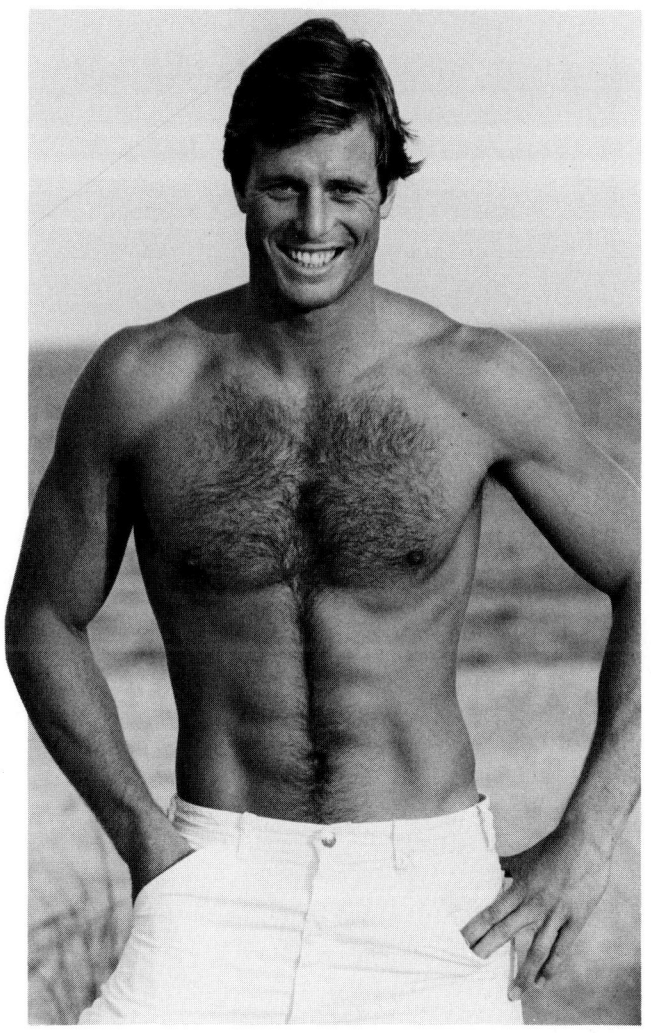

Rick Edwards
Vital & Not So Vital Statistics
Birthdate: August 8, 1955
Height: 6'1"
Weight: 170 lbs.
Hair: Dirty-blond
Eyes: Blue
Personal Favorites —
Town: Northfield, Massachusetts
Car: Shelby Cobra 427
Magazines: *Playboy; Auto Week*
Hero: "My dad"
Color: Red
Vacation Spots: Yosemite National Park; Big Sur, California
After-shave Lotion: Skin Bracer (Mennen)
Movie: *Butch Cassidy and the Sundance Kid*
Actors: Clint Eastwood; Paul Newman; Robert Redford
Actress: Katharine Hepburn
Authors: Robert Ludlum; James Clavell
Drink: Foster's Lager
Snack: Frozen seedless green grapes
Hobbies: Rowing; fast cars
Hangouts: Pete's Tavern, Metropolitan Cafe, Italian Trastevere, all in New York City
Goals: "I don't have enough time in my life to do everything I'd like, but I dream a lot."
Agency: Ford, New York City

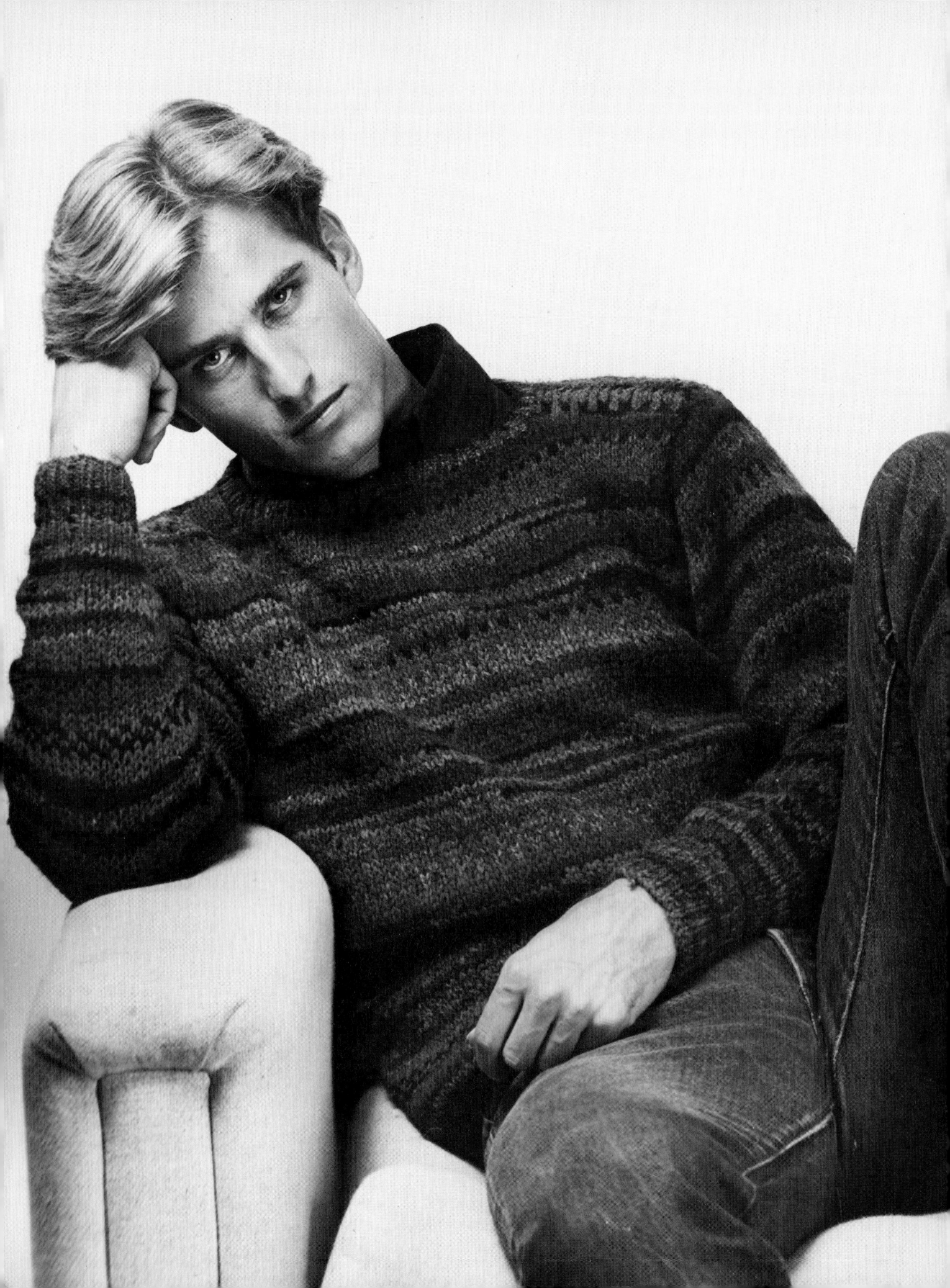

Michael Ives

If F. Scott Fitzgerald were still writing, he might well create a hero on the order of Michael Ives. Blond, blue-eyed, and blessed with a grin that suggests he's just scored the winning touchdown, Michael has enjoyed the charmed life of a Fitzgerald character. Born into a family of five boys in Glen Cove, New York, and educated at St. Paul's, an exclusive prep school in New Hampshire, Michael projects the Ivy League look. He is in fact a third-generation Yalie who graduated in 1979. An English major, Michael's favorite authors are D. H. Lawrence and John Donne; Michael says, "Donne is good. He's dirty." Still, Michael also enjoys action-packed novels and likes to imagine himself as an adventurer, like Luke Skywalker in *Star Wars*.

Michael Ives never envisioned a career as a model. Indeed, his career began with an accidental meeting that was a stroke of good luck. While spending the summer on Martha's Vineyard in 1974, he was stopped on the street one day by photographer Bruce Weber and asked to participate in a fashion spread for *GQ*. "At that point," says Michael, "I hadn't heard of Bruce Weber or *GQ*." But those photographs catapulted Michael into the world of modeling. He now appears regularly in high-exposure spreads, travels on assignment to Tunisia, Egypt, and Colombia, and has been on the cover of *GQ*. At twenty-five, he earns nearly one hundred thousand dollars a year.

Along with Jeff Aquilon, Michael was in part responsible for a dramatic change in men's fashion photography. Until Aquilon and Michael arrived, the prevailing pose was sophisticated and worldly. But Michael's easygoing, outgoing look triggered a revolution. "When I first came into the business, the look was not so all-American," recalls Michael. "It was more elegant. Now, the look is 'sportif.' I look very all-American — the California-sunshine, perpetually happy person. That's part of

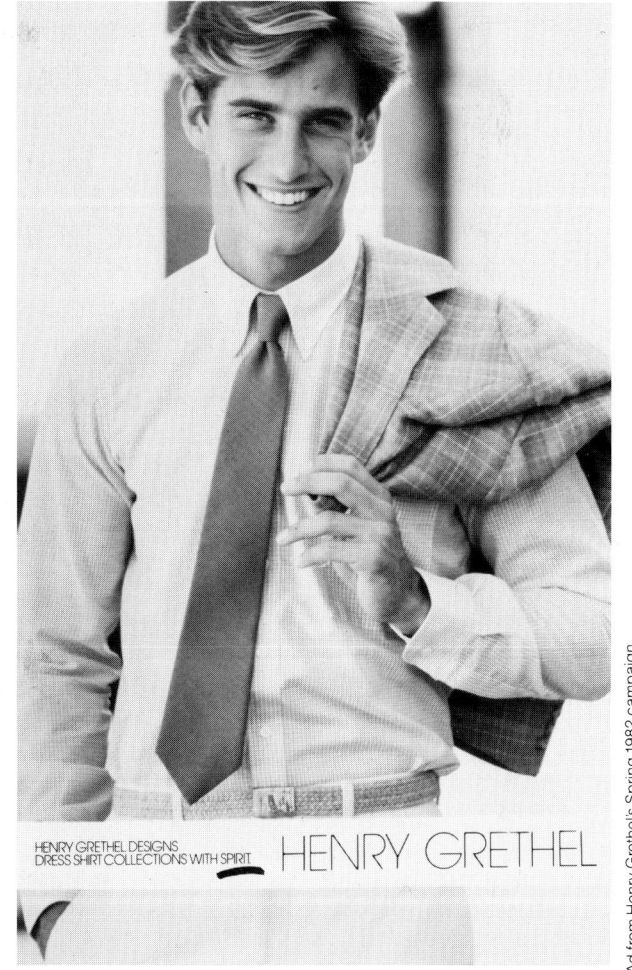

Ad from Henry Grethel's Spring 1982 campaign

17

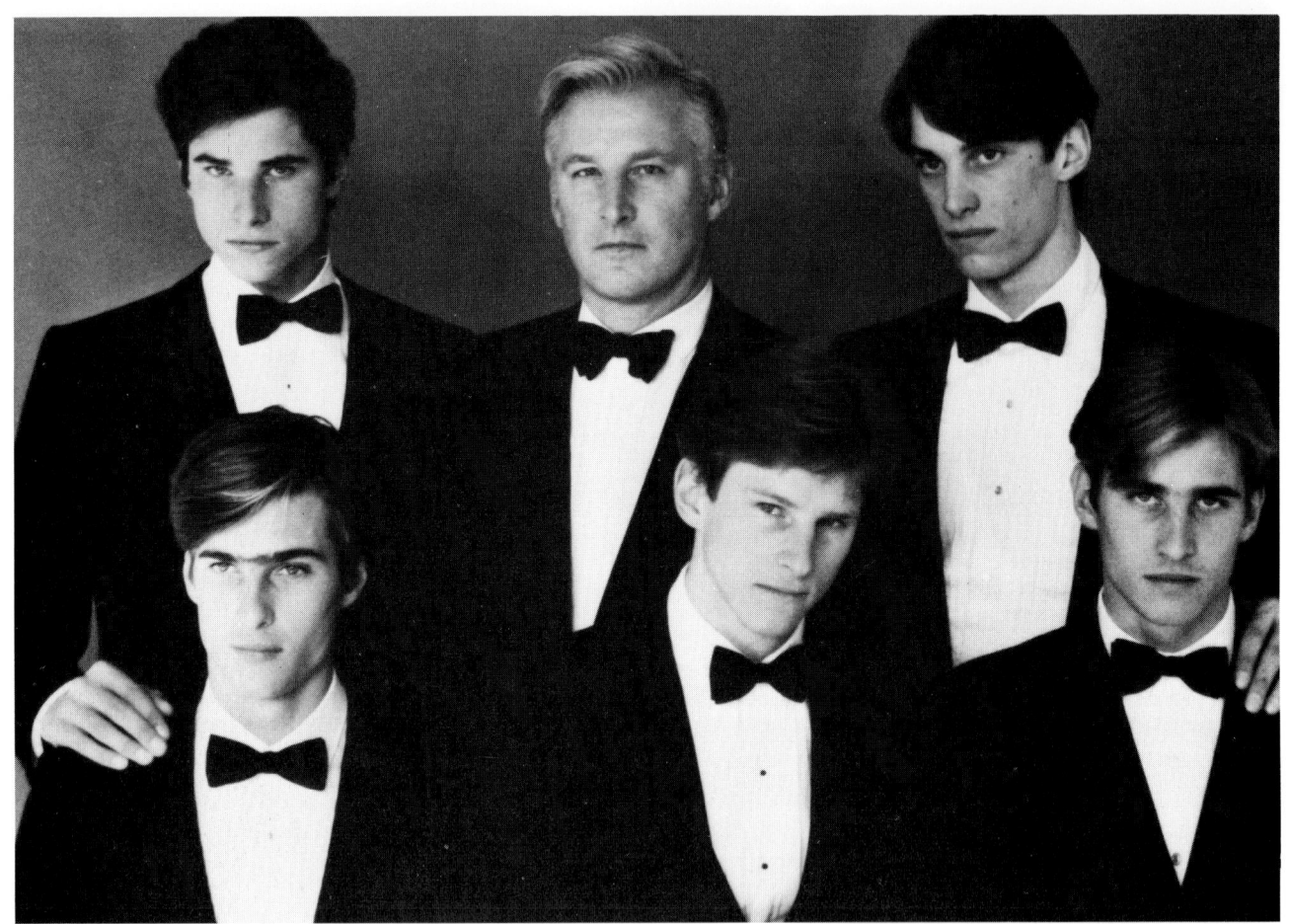

The Ives men: (top, l. to r.) George, Kenneth (father), Edward; (bottom, l. to r.) Chris, Ken, Michael.

the reason why I'm working. And that's fine with me. I'd rather be that type than in suits and tuxedos, because it's more the way I really am. My best pictures are when I'm just being myself."

Michael's reputation as an outdoor type is well-earned. For him, rowing is both a preoccupation and a family tradition. Two of his uncles were captains of Yale crew. "Rowing was a big part of why I was at Yale," he says. "I only applied to colleges where I could row." As a member of the Yale crew, Ives traveled around the country and to the Henley Regatta in England. He still has a drawer of highly prized T-shirts and trophies from his crew days. "Rowing is like a religion," he admits. "Girlfriends of rowers can never understand it."

Michael's boyish looks have earned him wide admiration. "The media has realized that men can be sexy, too, and that's opened a whole new market," he says. Although at first he found the attention unsettling, Michael has grown accustomed to fan mail and being stopped on the street by "somebody who knows me through somebody who knows somebody's daughter who is trying to be a model in Tennessee." Michael has maintained a level-headed attitude toward his early success, and his father, an investment banker in Boston, has kept a watchful eye on Michael's finances.

Michael's rise to fame has coincided with a new popularity for the preppie look. True to his own prep background and the look he has helped popularize, Michael usually dresses in "basic, functional, loose-fitting clothes" from Brooks Brothers and L. L. Bean. The consummate prep, he even prefers Brooks Brothers boxer shorts. Like many of his college classmates, Michael currently resides on the Upper East Side of New York, where he shares a two-bedroom apartment with his best friend from boarding school. The focal point of his living room is a Chickering piano, circa 1915 — purchased with some of his two-thousand-dollar-a-day modeling fees. But Michael spends as much time playing another object in the living room: an Atari game. Although he enjoys such luxuries, Michael is aware of the transitory nature of his work. "If I could give advice to anyone," he says, "it would be not to make modeling an exclusive thing. What modeling gives you is the financial freedom to do things that really matter to you in the long run."

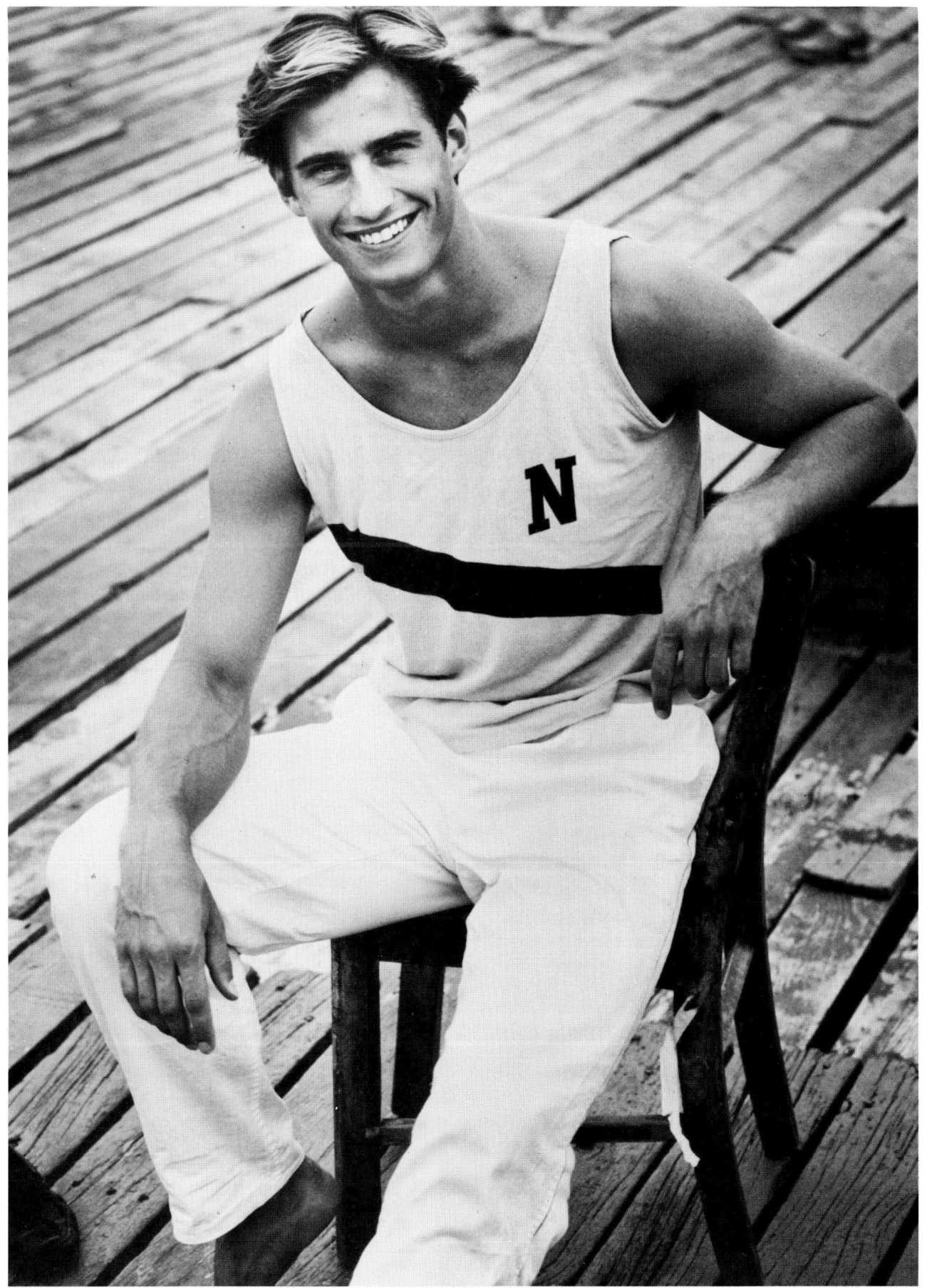

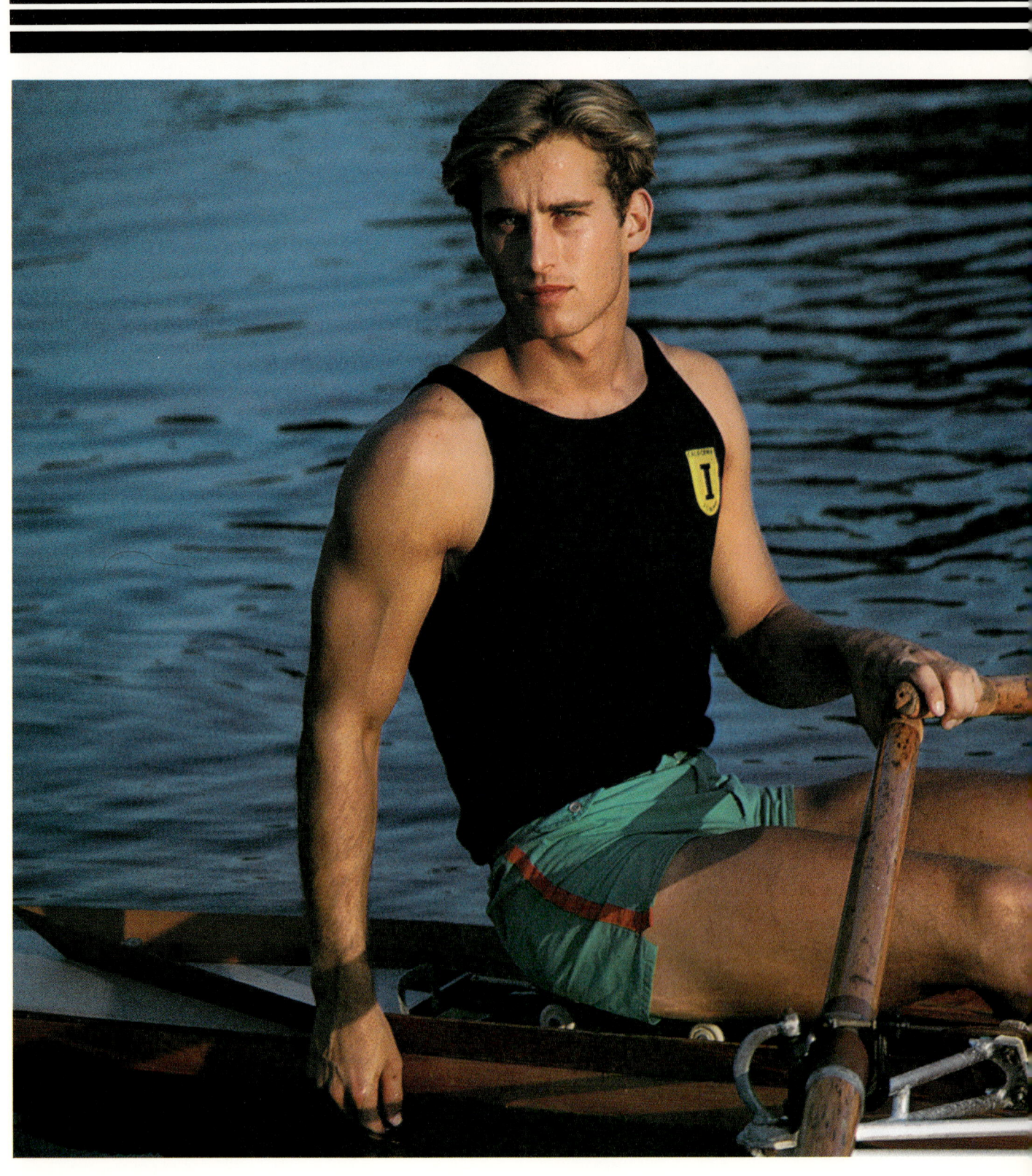

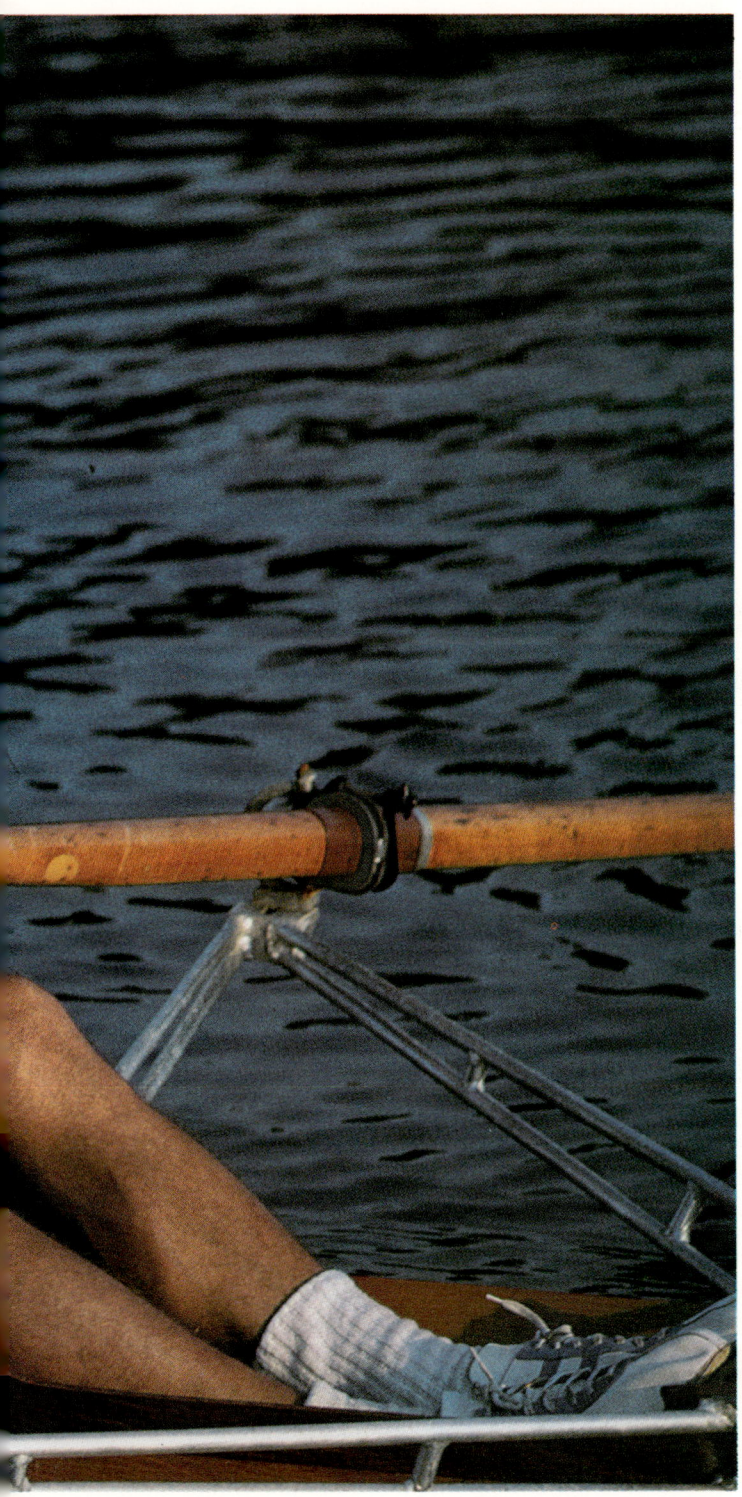

" I prefer a relationship when it's balanced. Sometimes I want to be aggressive and sometimes I want to be the passive one. Everybody has his moods. I would get very tired of a lopsided relationship, especially emotionally "

Michael Ives
Vital & Not So Vital Statistics
Birthdate: December 29, 1957
Height: 6'2"
Weight: 185 lbs.
Hair: Blond
Eyes: Blue

Personal Favorites —
Town: Dorset, Vermont
Snack: Drake's apple pies
Drink: Cranberry juice
Clothing Style: Brooks Brothers
Personal Hero: Underdog
Magazine: *National Geographic*
Hobbies: Playing the piano; soccer; skiing
Movie: *Raiders of the Lost Ark*
Actor: Alan Alda
Actress: Grace Kelly in *To Catch A Thief*
TV Show: *M*A*S*H*
Cartoon: *Bugs Bunny*
Music: Dan Fogelberg; Karla Bonoff
Hangouts: Oren and Aretsky, Jim McMullen's, both in New York City
Moisturizer: Aloe Vera Forever Tan
Agency: Wilhelmina, New York City

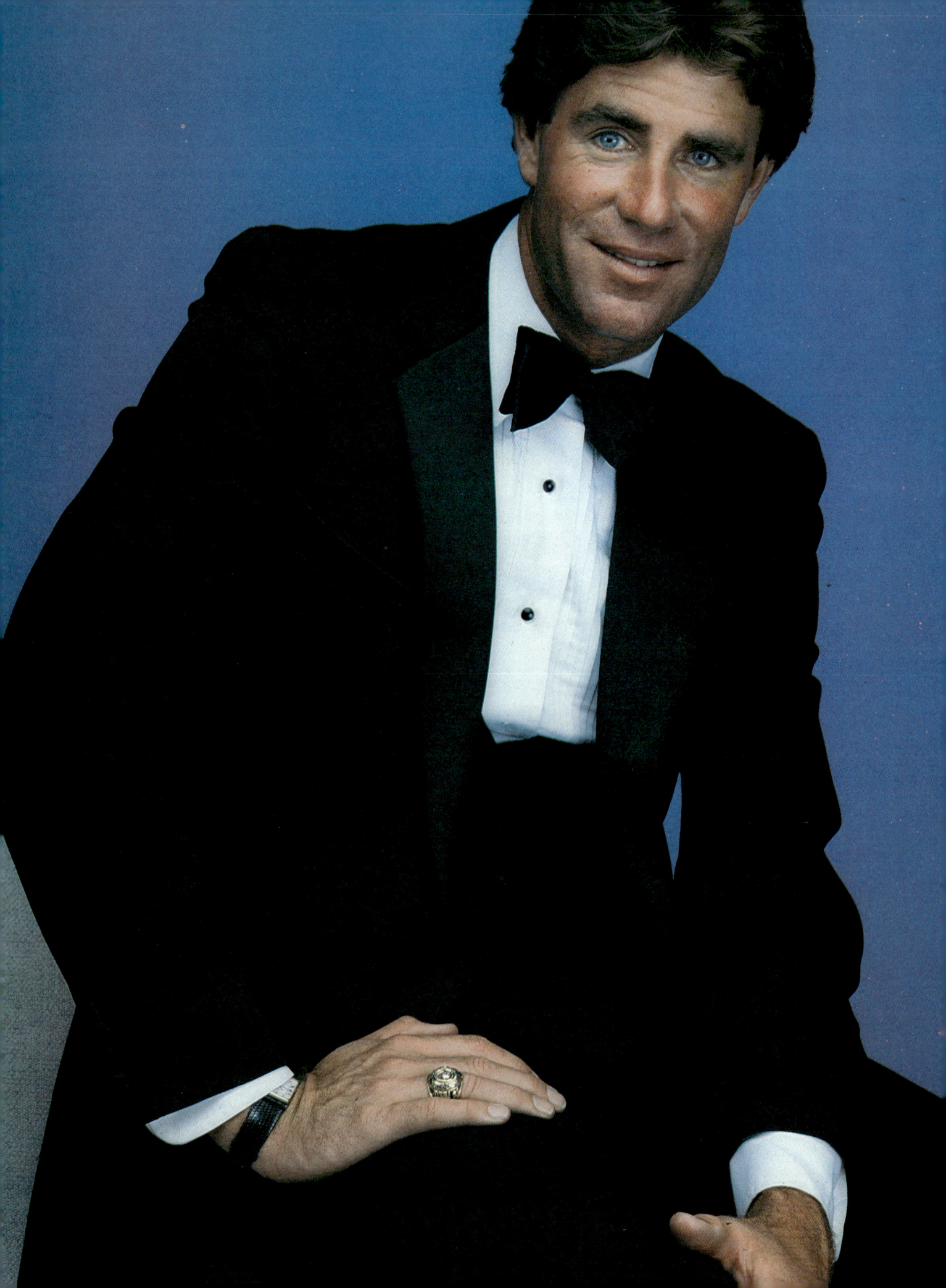

Jim Palmer

Jim Palmer may be one of the boys of summer, but he's a sex symbol for all seasons. His eighty-five-mile-per-hour fastball has made him immensely popular with baseball fans, and his mature, masculine looks have made him equally popular with women.

As a star of the Baltimore Orioles, Palmer is known for the fiery pitching that has won him three Cy Young awards. As the company spokesperson for Jockey International, Inc., he's known as the dashing figure in colored bikini briefs in Jockey ads. Jim's easygoing, good-natured manner makes him come across like the guy next door, but his baby-blue-eyed magnetism makes him stand out in the crowd. When Jim Palmer makes a personal appearance at a department store, hundreds of women stand in line for a signed color poster of him — self-assured, inviting, confident, and charismatic in a pair of Jockey Brand underwear. Jim Palmer is a classic American hero: a good sport on the field, a great guy off.

If modeling was an afterthought for Palmer, it has propelled him to the forefront of the public consciousness. "More people now know who I am," he says. And he admits, "It's very flattering to have somebody say that you look good in your underwear. It gives you a good feeling when you sign six hundred autographs in Kansas City."

Like numerous top models, Jim began his fashion career at someone else's suggestion. In 1976, executives of Jockey International invited Palmer to appear in a print ad with an all-star lineup of professional athletes, including Pete Rose, Steve Garvey, Tony Dorsett, and Steve Carlton. The ad asked: "Take away their uniforms, and who are they?" Three years later the brown-haired pitcher shut out his major-league competition and was chosen as the company's only spokesperson. "Of course I realize that if I didn't

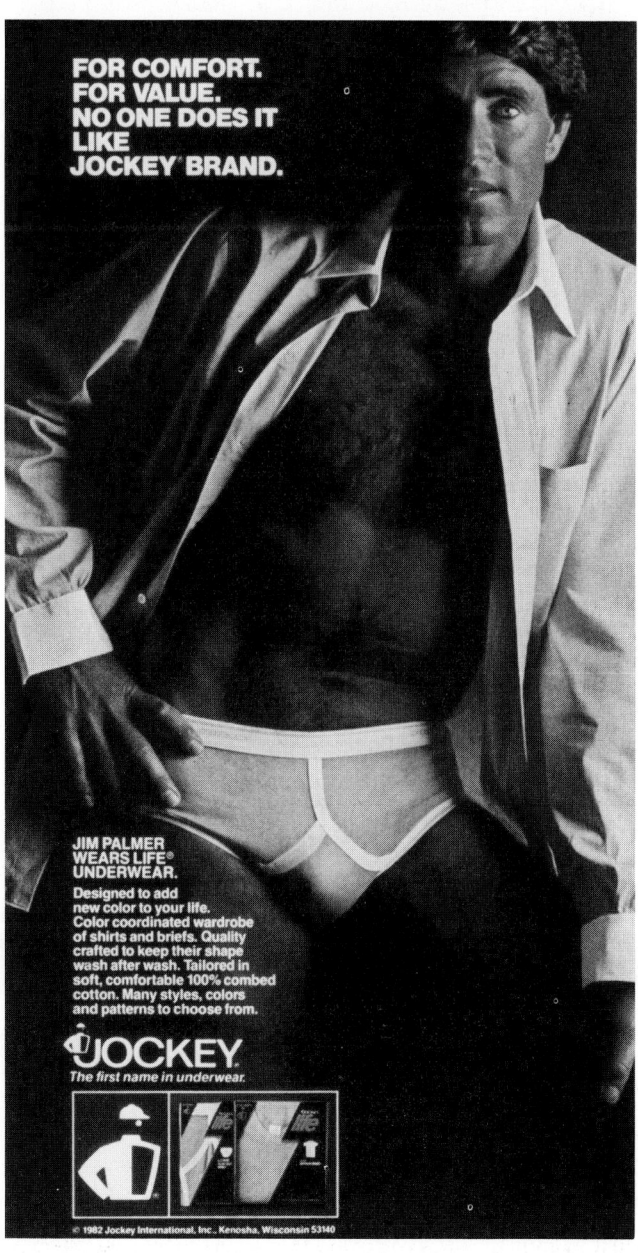

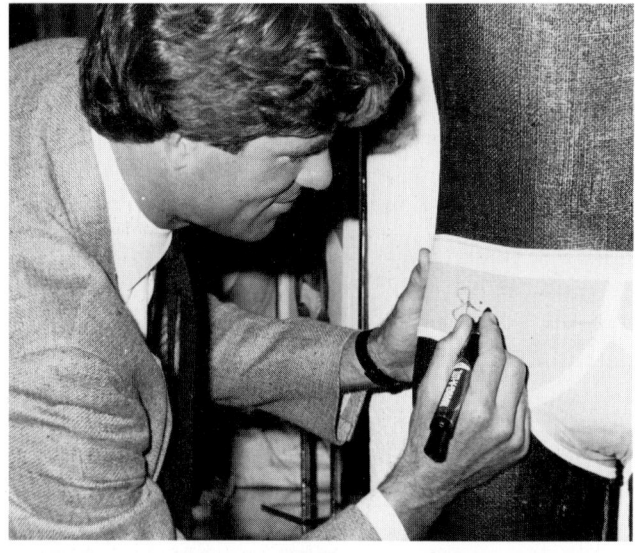
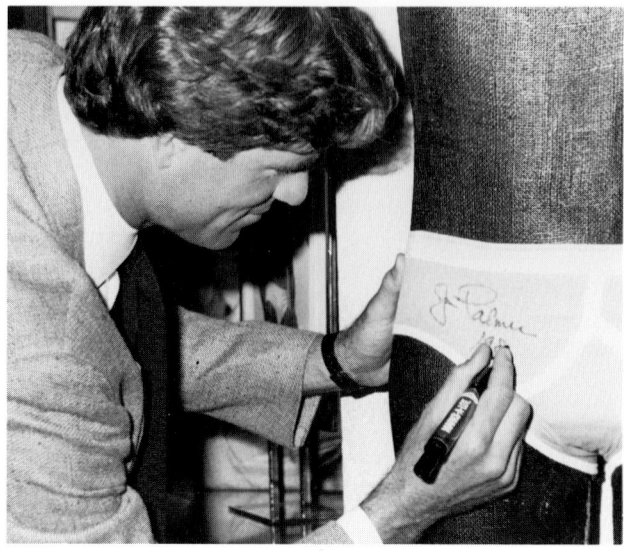
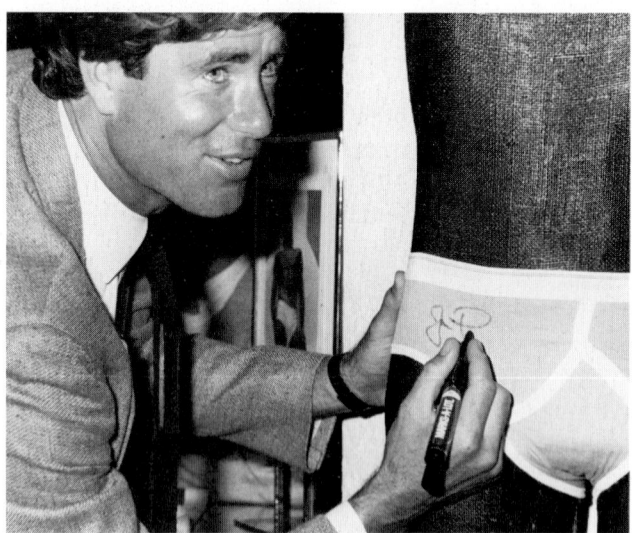

look good in their underwear or couldn't do the PR end of it, they would have hired somebody else."

Jim's poise has gotten him out of some awkward predicaments that his riveting good looks have gotten him into. During a promotional appearance in San Francisco, a female fan arrived wearing a pair of white Jockey Brand shorts over her black leotard. She asked Palmer to sign his name on the shorts across her derriere. Always the obliging gentleman, Jim complied. Still, Jim prefers to be known to his fans first and foremost for his considerable baseball accomplishments.

An adopted child, Jim spent his early years on Park Avenue in New York City, then moved with his family to Los Angeles and on to Scottsdale, Arizona, where he attended high school and earned varsity letters in football, basketball, and baseball. By the time he enrolled in Arizona State University, he was already being watched by scouts. He soon left college for a shot at the major leagues. Although he now lives in a suburb of Baltimore, Jim's heart is still in Arizona, judging from his home. The contemporary house has the southwestern charm and furnishings of an Arizona homestead. The living room boasts cathedral ceilings, exposed beams, and a massive stone fireplace. All around are oil paintings from Jim's extensive collection of southwestern art. He's the

James Arnold Palmer
Vital & Not So Vital Statistics
Birthdate: October 15, 1945
Height: 6'3"
Weight: 194 lbs.
Hair: Brown
Eyes: Blue
Personal Favorites —
Town: Boston
Time of Day: Dusk, "especially as the sun goes down"
Hangouts: The Great American Melting Pot, The Prime Rib Room, Alpine at the Belvedere Hotel, all in Baltimore; and Il Vagabondo, New York City
TV Show: *The Tonight Show* with Johnny Carson
Snack: Häagen-Dazs chocolate chocolate chip ice cream
Drink: Milk
Music: Frank Sinatra; Barbra Streisand; Bob James
Movie: *Play It Again, Sam*
Actors: Woody Allen; Robert Redford
Actress: Meryl Streep
Book: *The Fountainhead*
Authors: James Michener; Irving Wallace
Car: Silver Mercedes Turbo 300
Vacation Spots: Miami, Florida; Saint Croix, Virgin Islands
Magazines: *Time; Newsweek; Esquire; The New Yorker*
Designer: Pierre Cardin
After-shave Lotion: Pierre Cardin
Hobbies: Tennis; racquetball; theater; landscaping the backyard
Hero: John Wayne

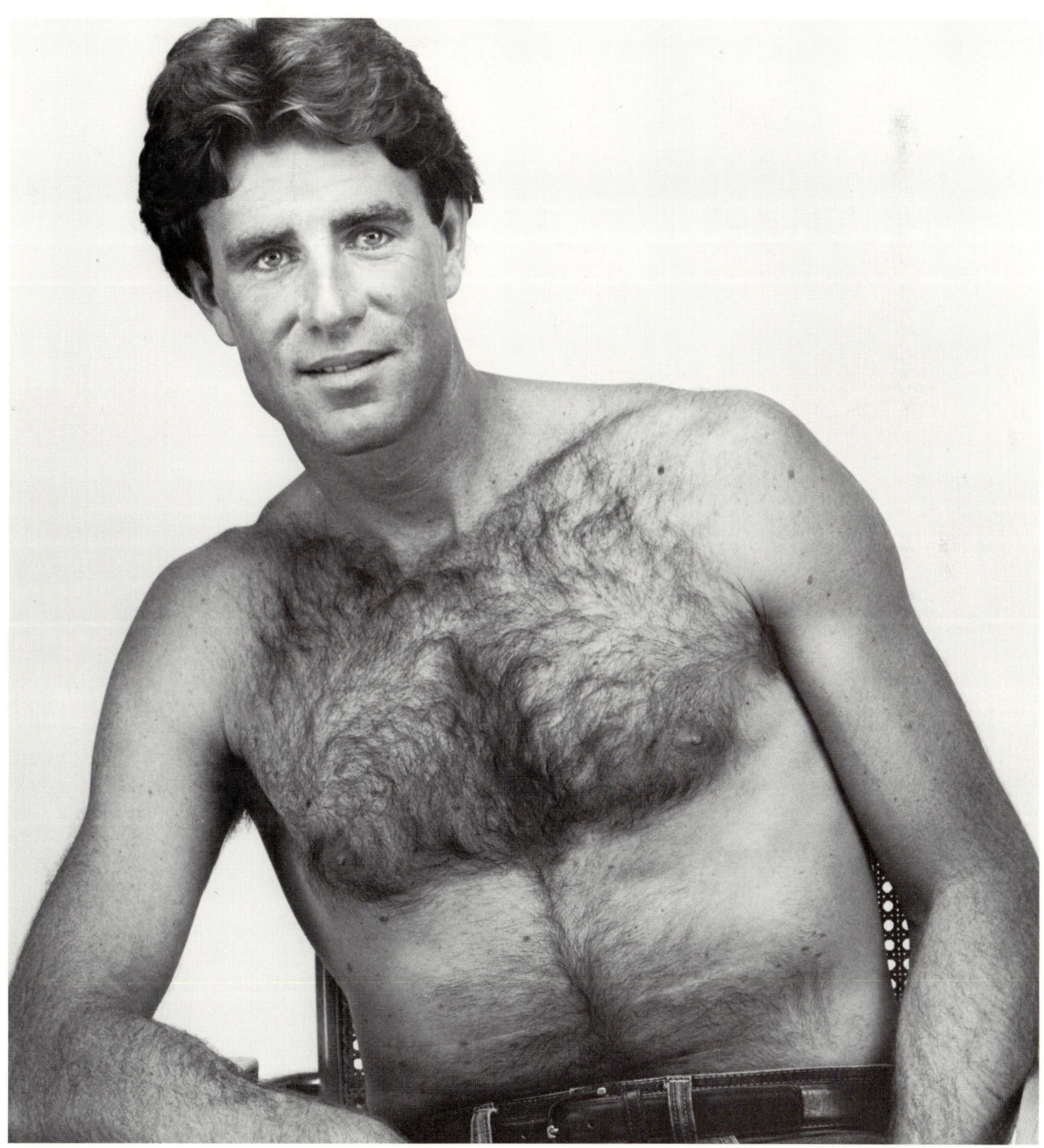

devoted father of two teenage daughters, Jamie and Kelly, with whom he tries to spend as much time as possible.

Surely bound for baseball's Hall of Fame, Jim has also set his sights on a much sought after but seldom attained prize for pro pitchers: three hundred lifetime wins. With that goal still a few seasons away, Jim says, "Not too many people win that many. All you try to do is be consistent. You just prepare yourself and try to do your best." After baseball, Jim may move full-time into television, where he has already provided commentary for ABC-TV during the World Series and other events.

Whatever the future holds, Jim Palmer isn't likely to shed his sex-symbol image. "I try to take care of myself for a number of reasons," he says. "It's silly not to take full advantage of the talent God gave you. I've seen too many athletes who have had their careers cut short by total disregard for their well-being. I would hate to look back at my career and say, 'If only I had taken care of myself, I could have been better.'"

Incidentally, does Jim Palmer wear Jockey Brand underwear himself? "Of course."

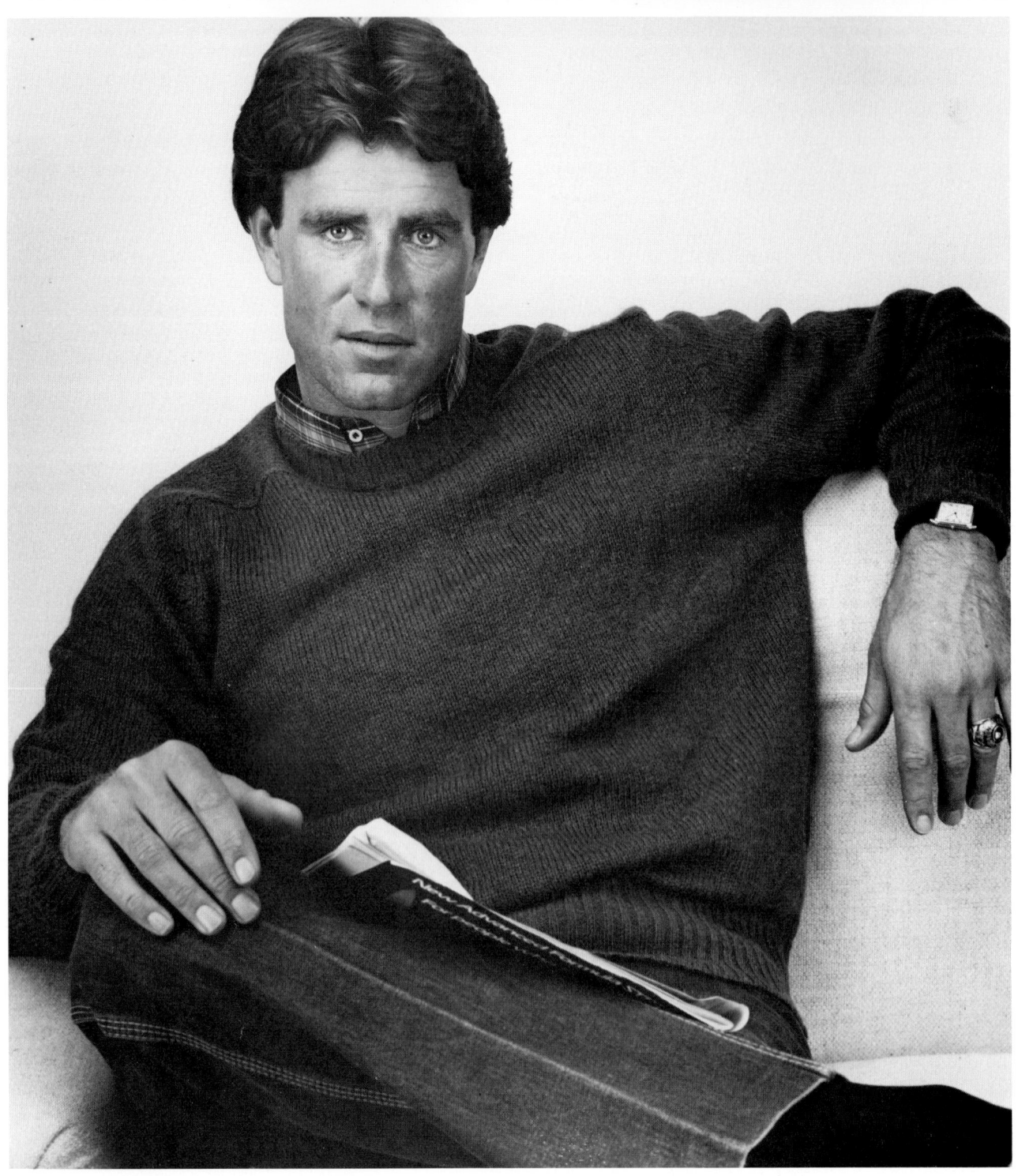

"My lifestyle is such that I can dress casually, but I also dress conservatively. I feel just as comfortable in a clean pair of jeans and a shirt as I do in a suit."

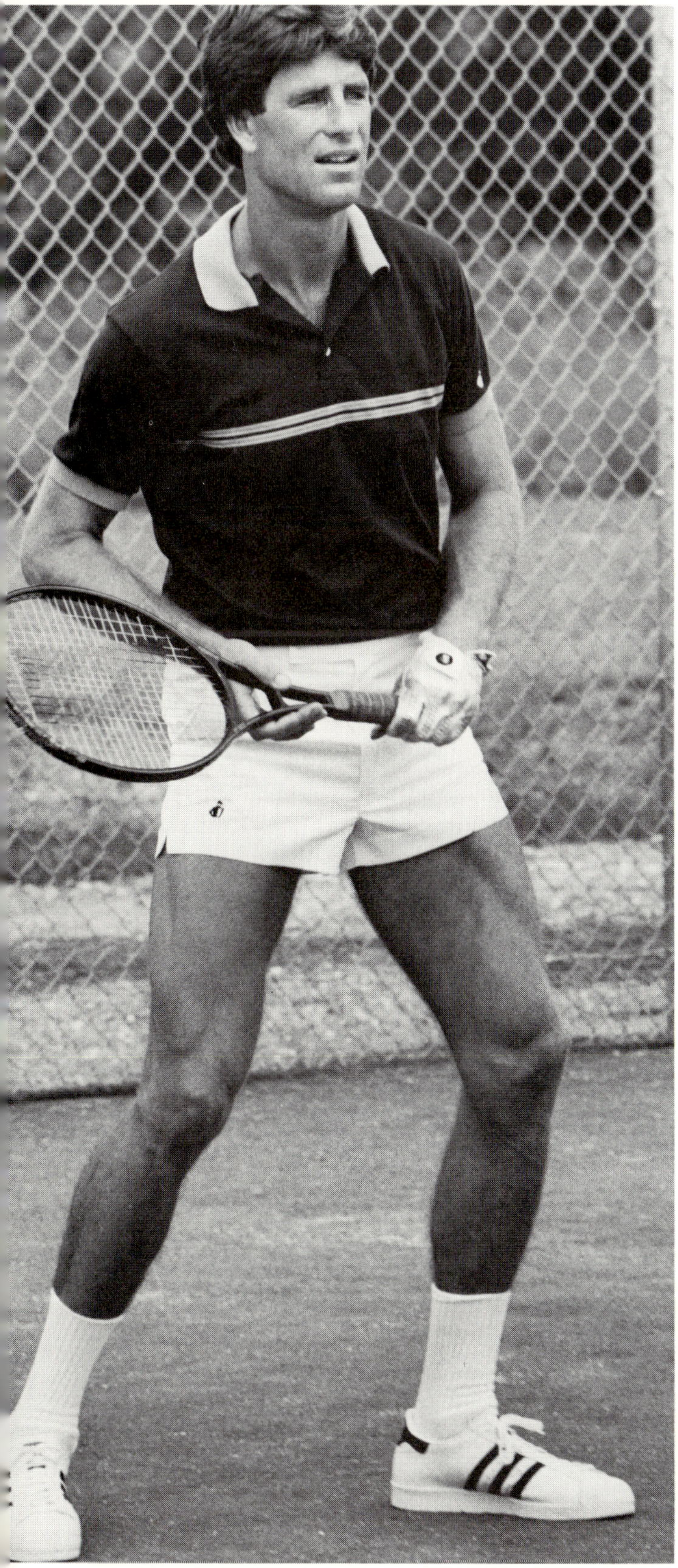

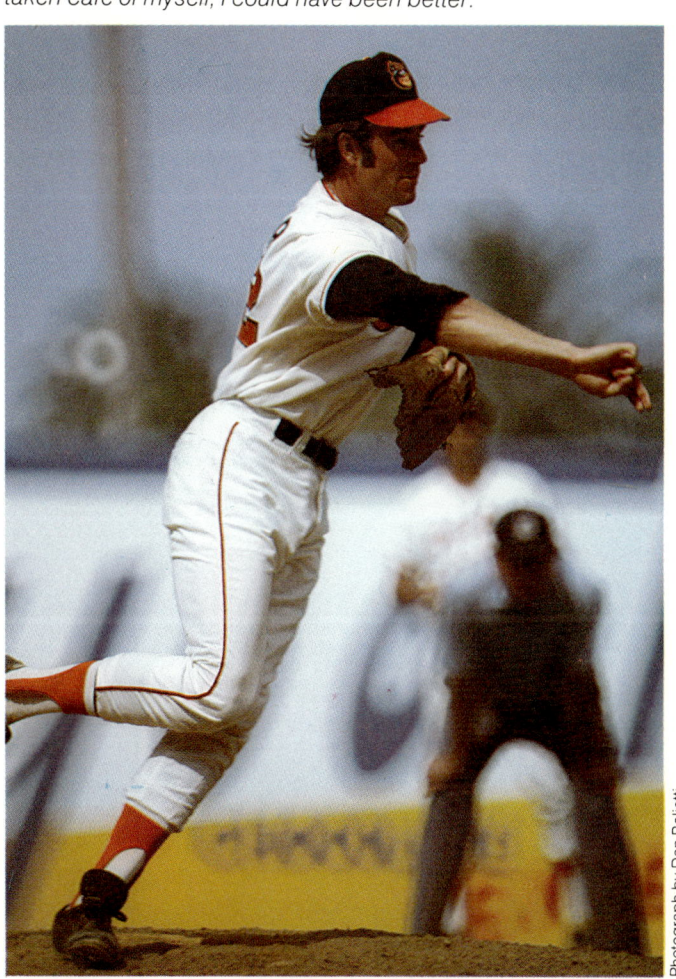

"I would hate to look back on my career and say, 'If only I had taken care of myself, I could have been better.'"

Photograph by Dan Baliotti

Over the years,
you realize that in baseball,
you're a hero
when you win and
a bum when you lose

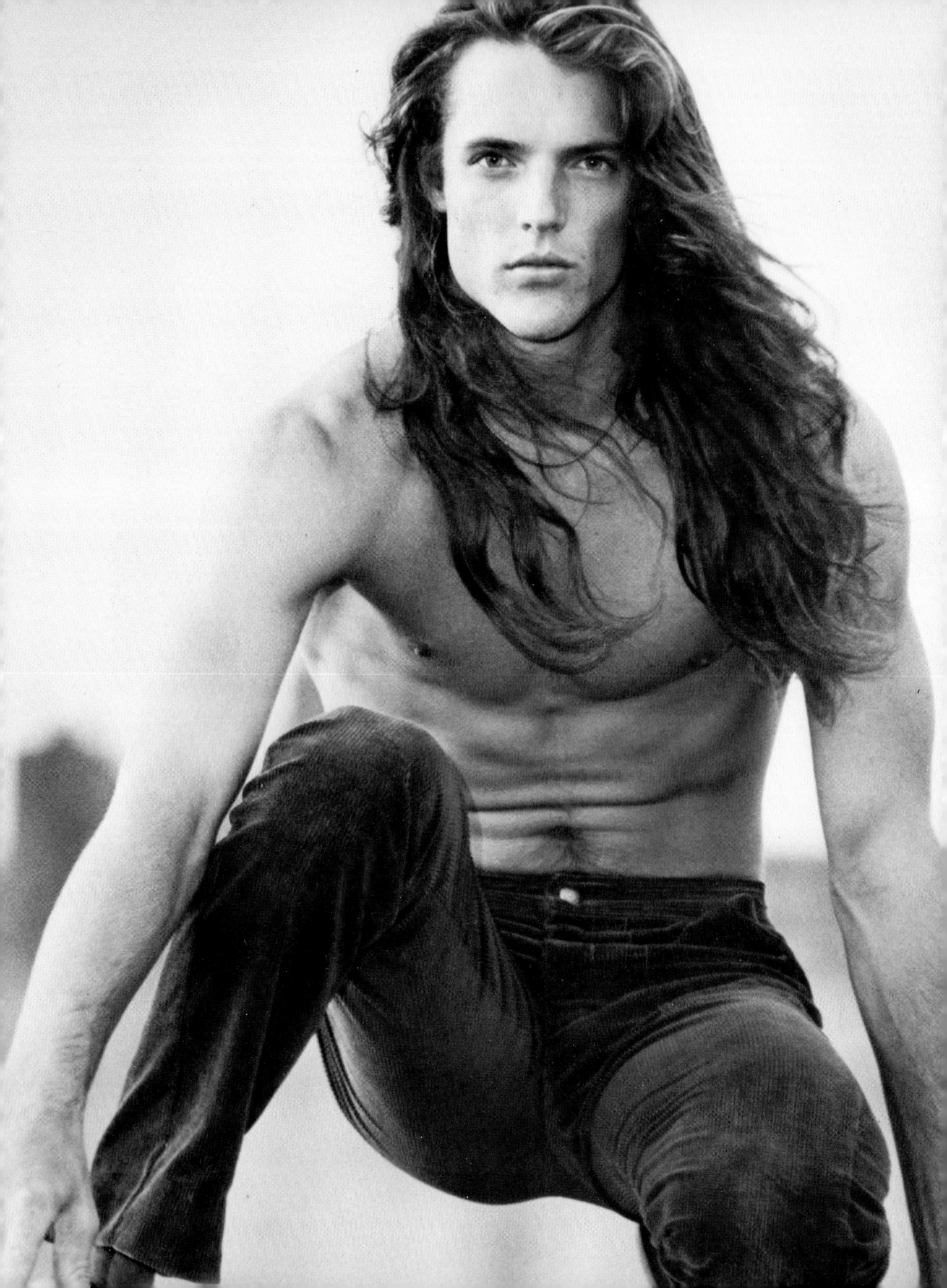

Attila Von Somogyi

His name is Attila Von Somogyi, but he's known in the trade as Attila the Hunk. Tall, solidly built, and just entering his twenties, Attila is one of the youngest successes in modeling. To some observers, his long locks make him look like a male version of Brooke Shields, but everyone agrees that Attila is a unique combination of sun-kissed California athleticism and exotic European features.

Attila has an unusual background to match his unusual name. (The youngest of three, he has a brother named Zoltan and a sister named Ildico.) His parents were wealthy Hungarian landowners who became partisan fighters when World War II broke out. According to Attila, the "Von" in his name was a title bestowed long ago, and "Somogyi" is the name of a county. "My family goes back probably seven hundred years in recorded history," he says. Although his parents didn't speak English when they came to this country, they settled in California and quickly assimilated. Attila's father became a fencing and soccer coach at the University of California in Santa Barbara and Attila himself began to indulge in beach sports. "Surfing is really a big part of my life," he says. "I couldn't live without it. I just love it. I've been doing it for about seven years now."

Attila got into modeling as a result of an unusual day at the beach. He recalls, "I was down at the beach with my ex-girlfriend. She was moving to Hawaii, and she'd hired a photographer to get some portrait shots of us, so she'd have shots to remember us by. Bruce Weber was down there doing a shoot, and he kept looking over, trying to figure out what was going on. He wasn't used to someone with long hair. We started to talk, and he asked me if I'd like to work, and the next day we did a shoot together."

Appropriately, those first photographs made exceptional use of Attila's shoulder-length brown

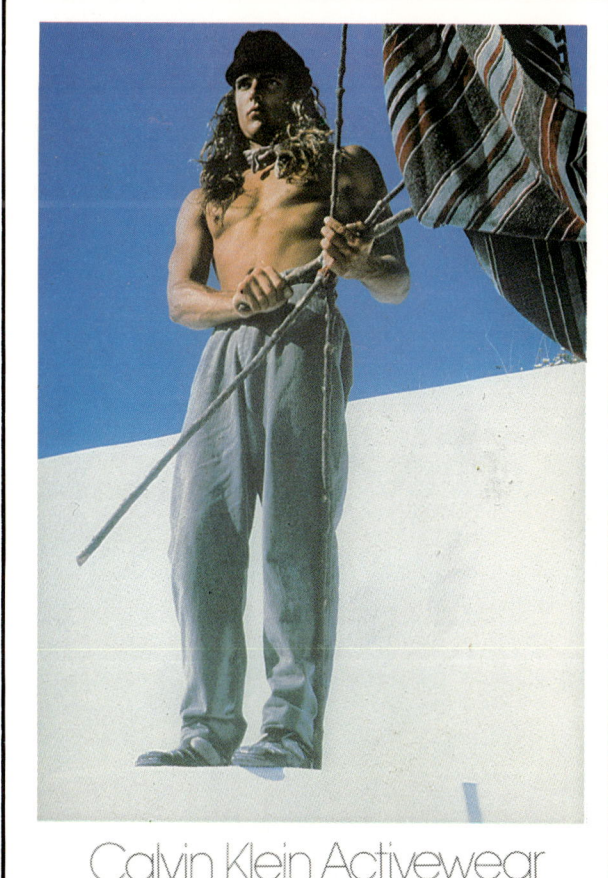

Calvin Klein Activewear

Attila Von Somogyi wearing Calvin Klein Activewear photographed by Bruce Weber

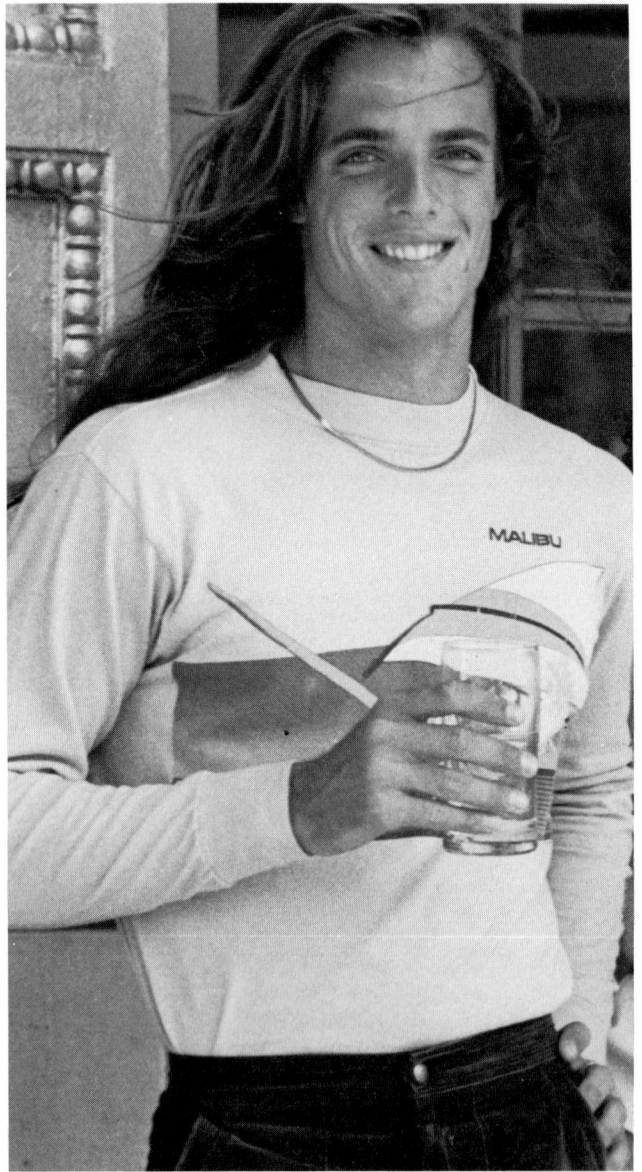

"On a regular day, I wake up, get breakfast, take a shower, and call up some of my friends. We either go to the beach or the mountains. At night, we go to parties and just generally have a lot of fun."

hair: the advertisement was for a Vidal Sassoon grooming product. Soon after, Calvin Klein noticed Attila. "I was flown out to New York, and I got to meet him, and I tried on some clothes," says Attila. "It's funny, because I didn't have any pictures, so I showed them my high school ID and driver's license. Those were the only pictures I had." Although relatively inexperienced, Attila got the job and was next flown to Greece for a Klein shoot. Attila's relaxed demeanor in front of a camera comes naturally. "I don't mind standing in front of a camera and taking pictures," he says. "It's like a paid vacation."

Attila's long hair distinguishes him as a novelty among models, and he treats it with the special care and respect accorded a prize possession. He conditions it after every shampoo "because it would take forever to comb out if I didn't," Attila adds. "I've had shoulder-length hair since about seventh grade. It's always been a kind of a trademark of mine in Santa Barbara. I like my hair long. It's part of me. If I happened to wake up one morning and my hair was short, it would be a nightmare. I'd just go nuts and smash everything in the room. I think hair is really great." Attila's favorite is Head shampoo. "It doesn't pollute the environment, and it makes your hair really soft and silky."

As befits a fellow with shoulder-length hair, Attila harbors a desire to succeed as a rock musician. He performed with a band in high school, singing lead vocals and playing guitar. "That's one of my biggest dreams, to be a rock star. What I'd really like to do is move to New York and get a vocal coach, because there are no good vocal coaches in California. They're just really into money."

Although his hair makes him resemble one of the bad boys in a rock-and-roll band, Attila's life-style is as American as apple pie. He lives at home with his mother ("we're best friends") and brother. He drinks a gallon of milk a day, he estimates. To stay in shape, he says, "I just stay active: sports, surfing, hiking. If you sit around and do nothing, you'll just deteriorate." And Attila's fashion sense is as fresh and relaxed as he is himself. "I usually don't really get too dressed up. I wear shorts, corduroys, a nice shirt, whatever. I dress casual. I've never worn a tie. I'd like to, though. I think it'd be fun."

Attila Von Somogyi
Vital & Not So Vital Statistics
Birthdate: June 3, 1963
Height: 6'
Weight: 165 lbs.
Hair: Brown
Eyes: Green
Personal Favorites —
Color: Purple-blue
Snack: Milk – "At my house a gallon will disappear in a day."
TV Shows: Saturday Night Live; SCTV
Music: Hard rock – Deep Purple; Led Zeppelin
Vocal Musicians: Ronny-James Diot; Steve Perry
Hobbies: Singing; surfing; hiking; cooking crepes; camping
Hair Products: Head shampoo and cream rinse
Ambition: "To be a rock star"
Designer: Calvin Klein
Moisturizer: Oil of Olay
Car: Black Lamborghini with tinted windows
Vacation Spot: Greek Islands
Ice Cream: Rocky road
Agency: Click, New York City

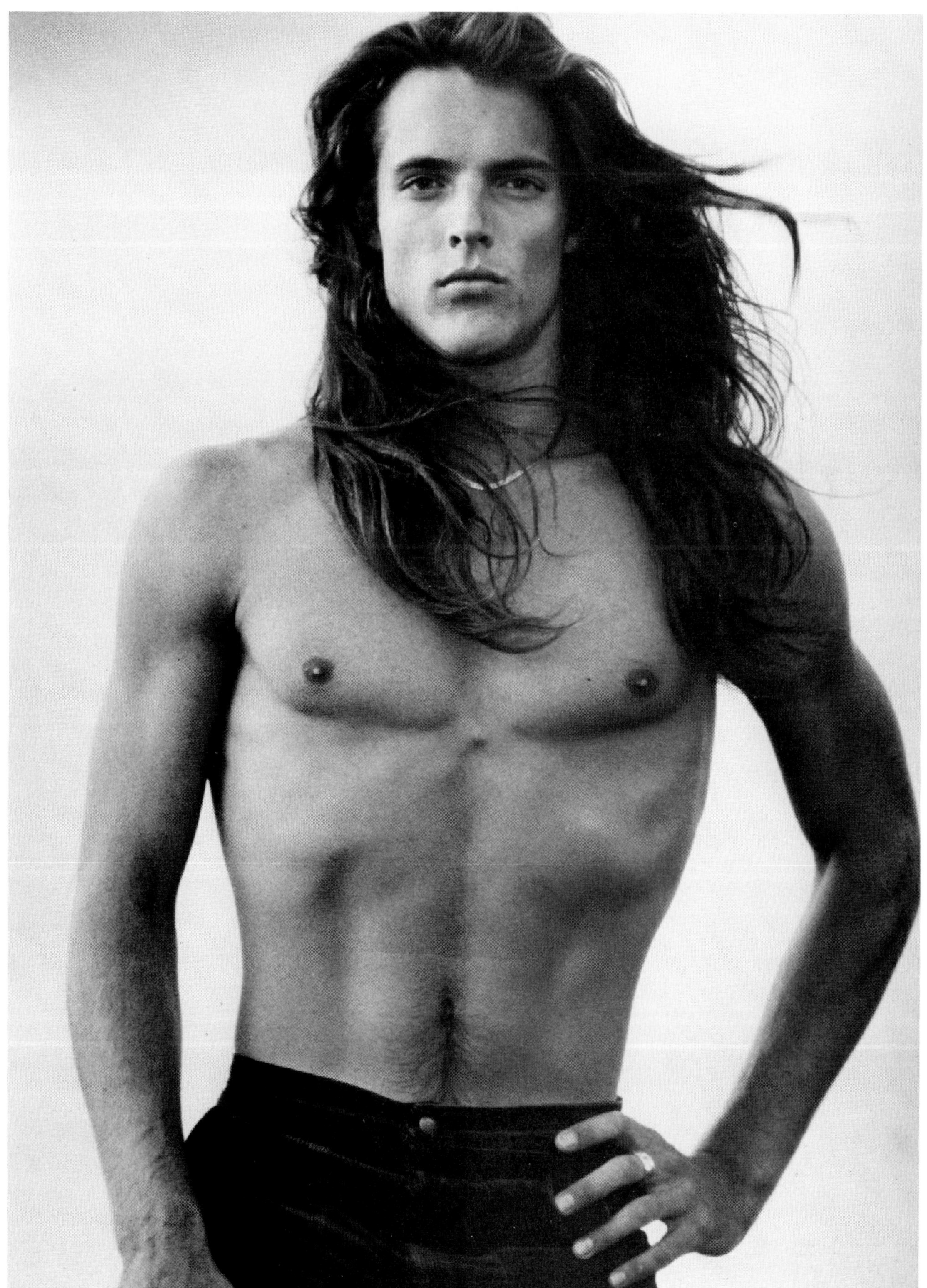

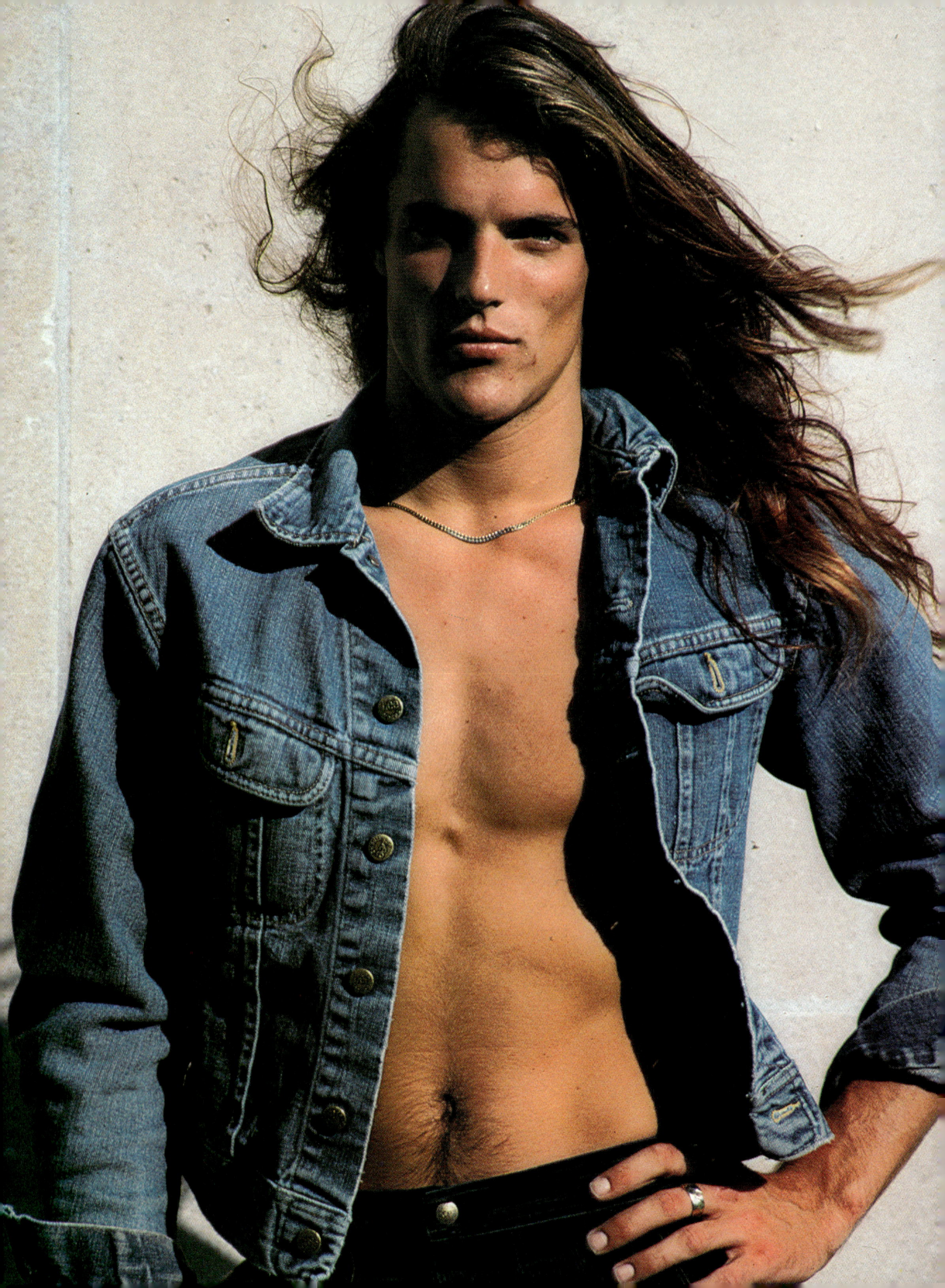

❛
I've got this obsession with being successful.
I *have* to be successful. Just to have a lot of money so I can support myself and not have to worry about a lot of things. That's life.
❜

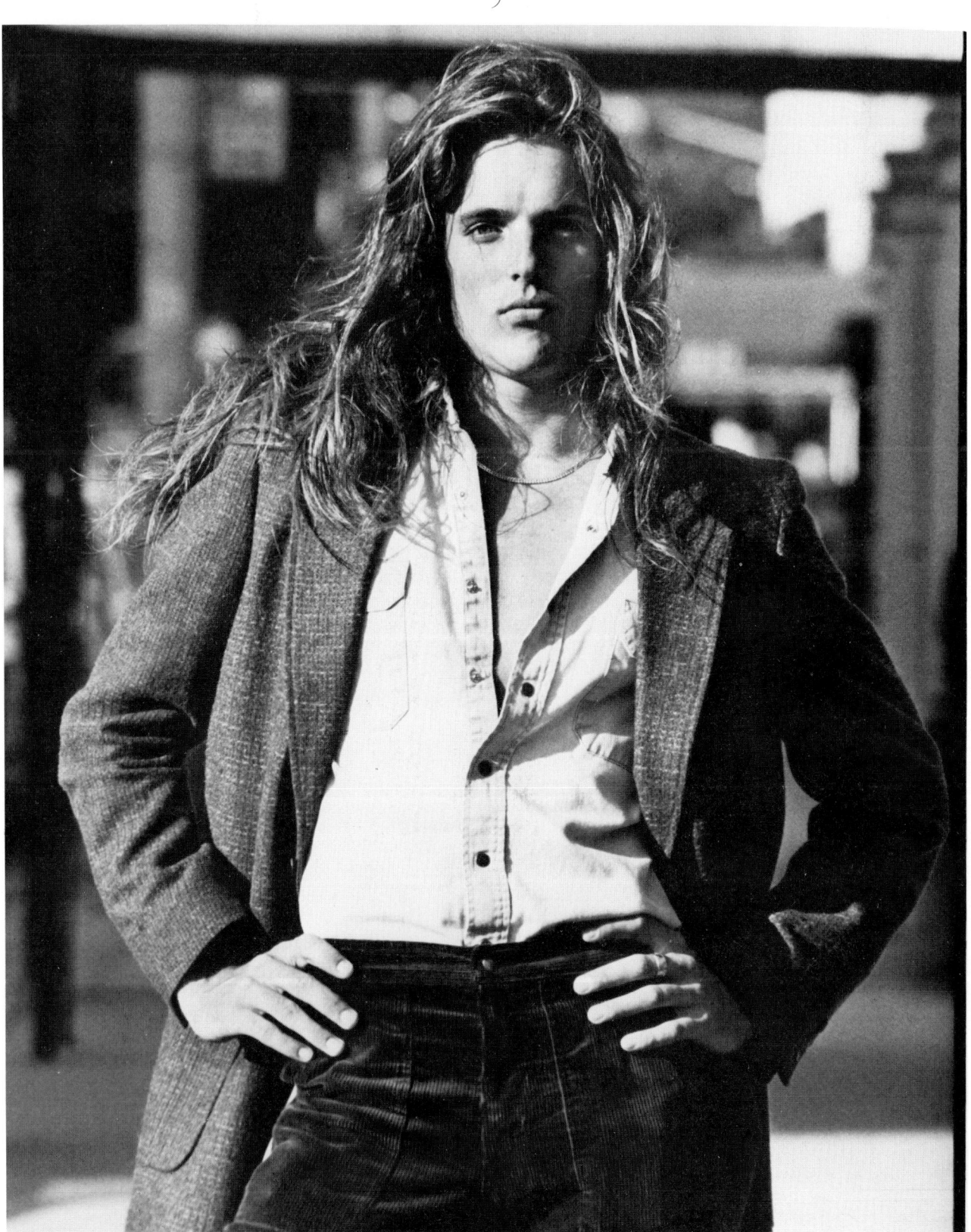

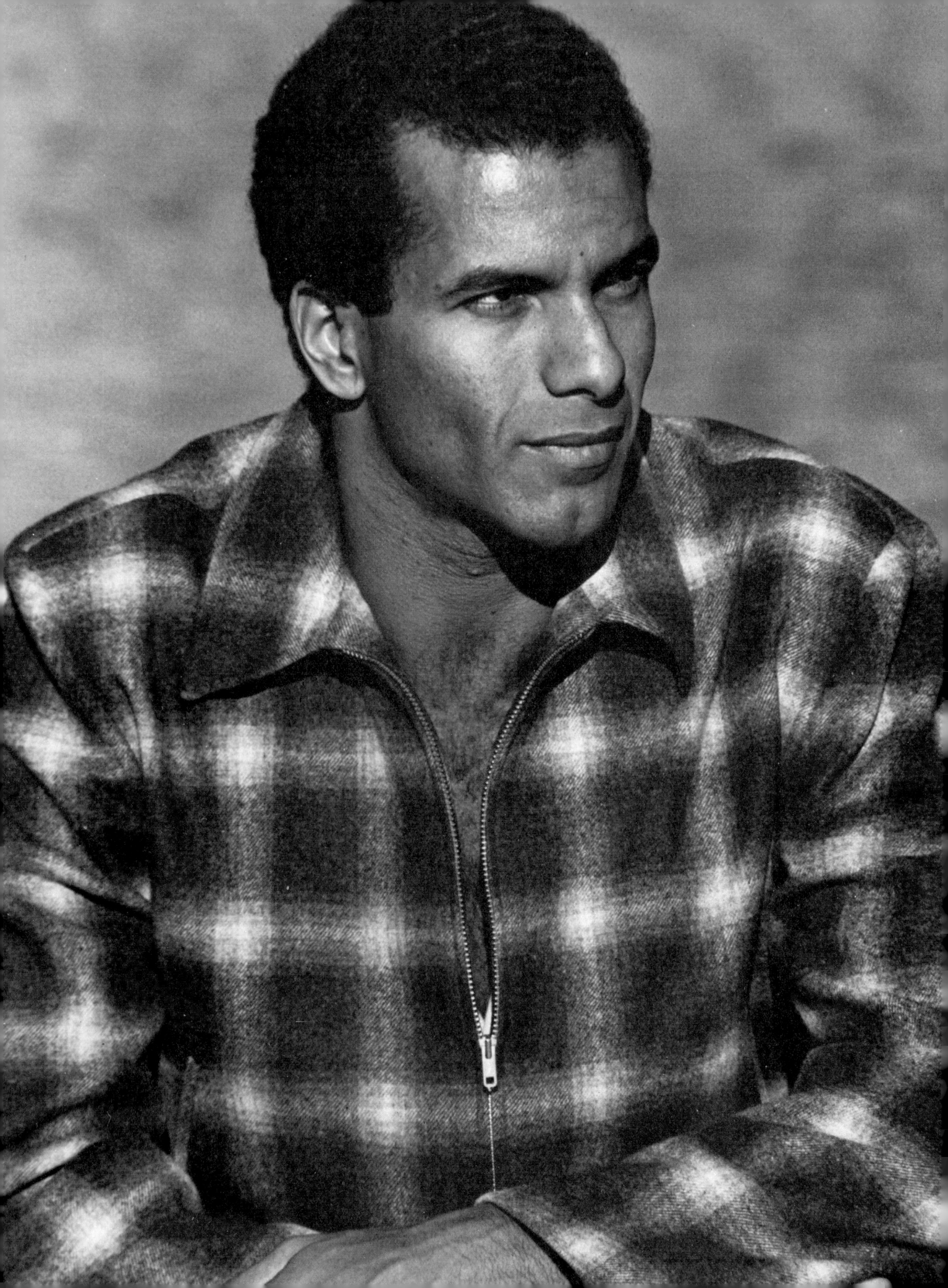

Charles Williamson

Charles Williamson has worked in the fashion world longer than some of the designers whose clothes he models. Charles is one of the few black male superstars in fashion, but his has been a long, difficult climb to the top. After a decade in the business, he's one of its most seasoned — and most persistent — veterans. It took Charles, for instance, ten years to receive a *GQ* cover. In an industry in which stars often burn out as quickly as they rise, Charles's longevity is a testament to the sometimes slow rewards of a fast-paced business. "Sometimes I ask myself why I stuck it out," he says. "Well, once I start something, I like to finish it. Looking back, it's taught me a lot above and beyond the business. I didn't work a lot at first, which gave me time to discover myself. That's the most important thing to me. That's probably the real reason why I stuck it out."

In his pictures, Charles's strikingly handsome face and poised demeanor epitomize a smiling success story; he looks like the dapper, confident leader. "Most of my pictures are smiling rather than aloof and macho," he notes. "I like that. It makes me more of a human being instead of some *thing* or object." But Charles believes his looks transcend categorization, particularly the category of *black* model. "I don't feel I project an image," he says. "I'd rather be me, and have nothing, than present an image and lose me."

Charles puts a high premium on individuality. "The most important thing in my life is my personal growth. Everything else should be an aid to that." That search has taken Charles across the continent. Born in Grenada, British West Indies, he came to the United States when he was eight. After high school, he worked as a bonds clerk on Wall Street. Drafted into the armed services, he entered the Marine Corps at age nineteen. "That was total chaos," he says. "I hated it. I had the worst time. The way they treat you is completely inhuman."

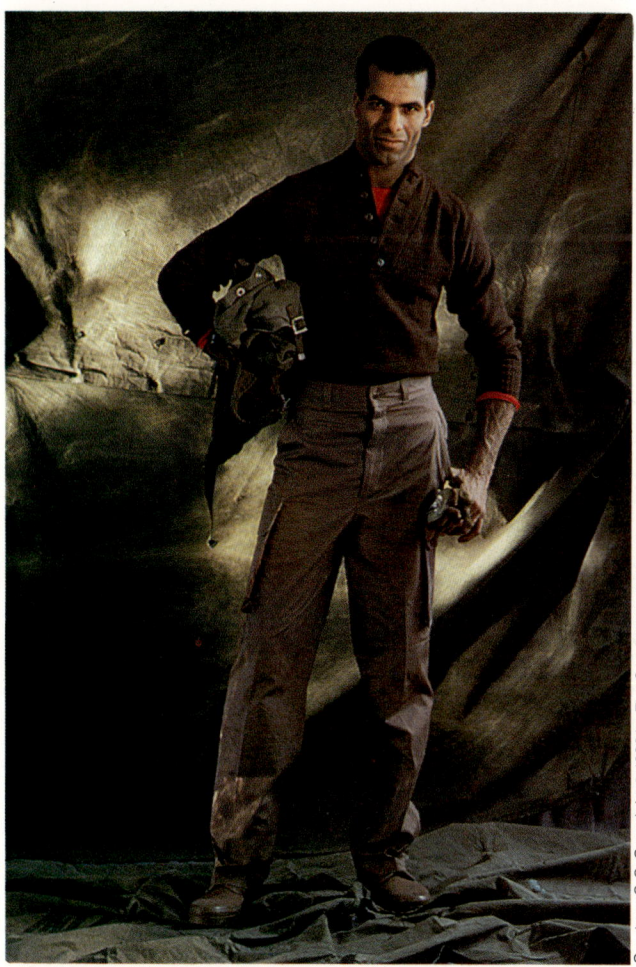

Courtesy G.Q. Copyright © 1982 by The Condé Nast Publications Inc.

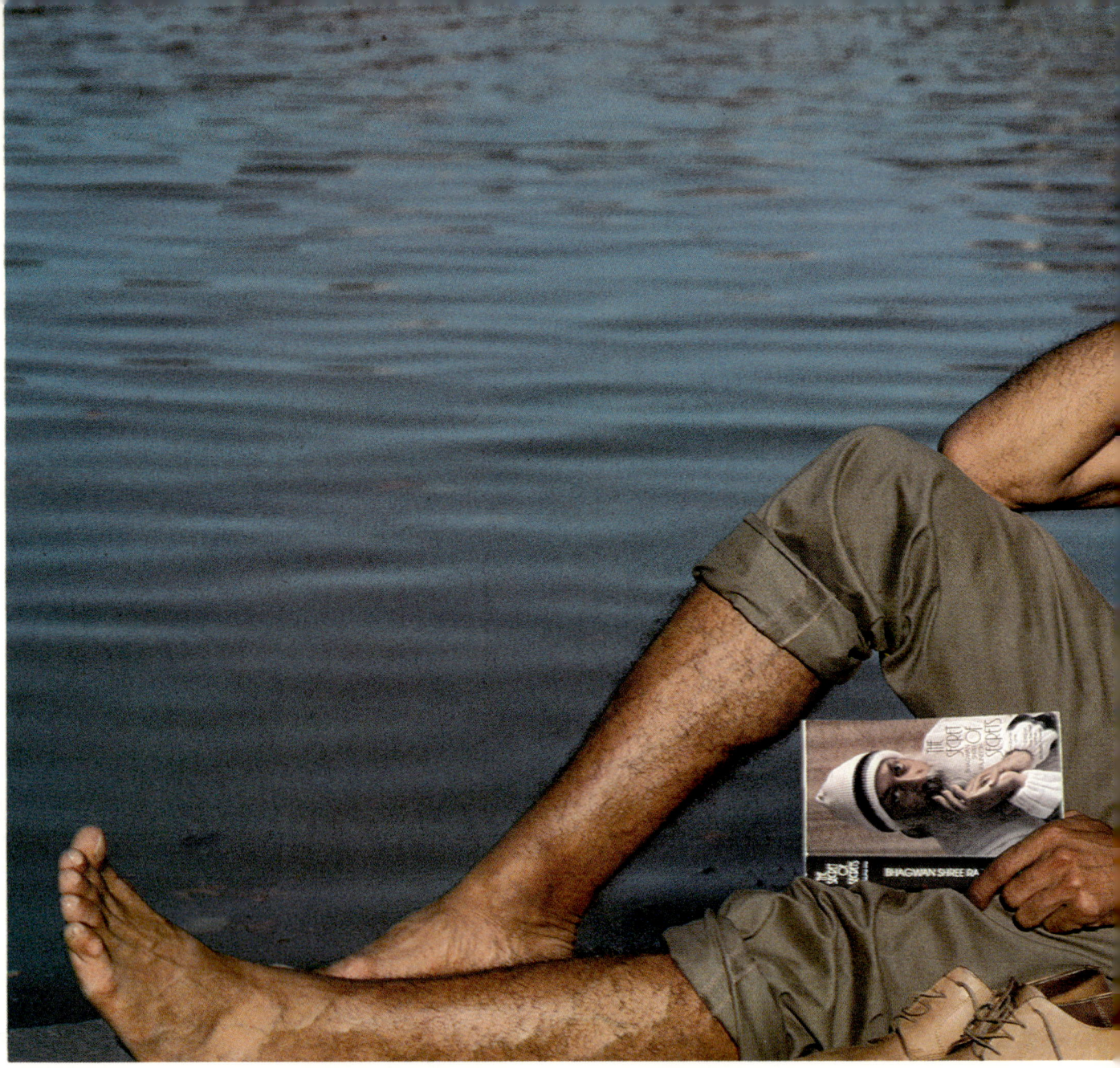

After the Marines, he returned to New York, where he maintains an apartment on the West Side. He also returned to Wall Street — briefly. "To me, it was just not worth getting ulcers to make money," he says, so he decided to try modeling at the urging of several friends.

At first, Charles worked with an agency called Black Beauty, but as a black man in a white-dominated industry, he saw a side of the business that wasn't always beautiful. His cheerful countenance and relaxed manner camouflage the difficulties initially encountered. "In terms of advertising dollars, black male models are at the bottom on the totem pole," he observes. "There's just not as much work. Black men aren't always used, even when they could be. Racism still exists in this industry. If I wanted to carry a chip on my shoulder, I could get very angry."

Instead, Charles believes that questions of race must be superseded. When he started modeling, he says, "I was told that I was too good looking, that I wasn't black enough, or that I wasn't white enough." As Charles sees the issue, "It's not about whether you're black or white. It's about you as an individual. I'm just as good or better than any other male model in the business, and I won't compromise. You lose yourself by compromising. This business is nothing but politics, and those who claim otherwise probably play the most." As someone who has forged his success his way, Charles is uncomfortable with the notion that he is a role model for young blacks entering the business. "I don't feel like a star," he says. "Behind here, I'm just a regular guy. I don't believe in people trying to be like somebody else. You're on the wrong track then. You're headed for failure right away."

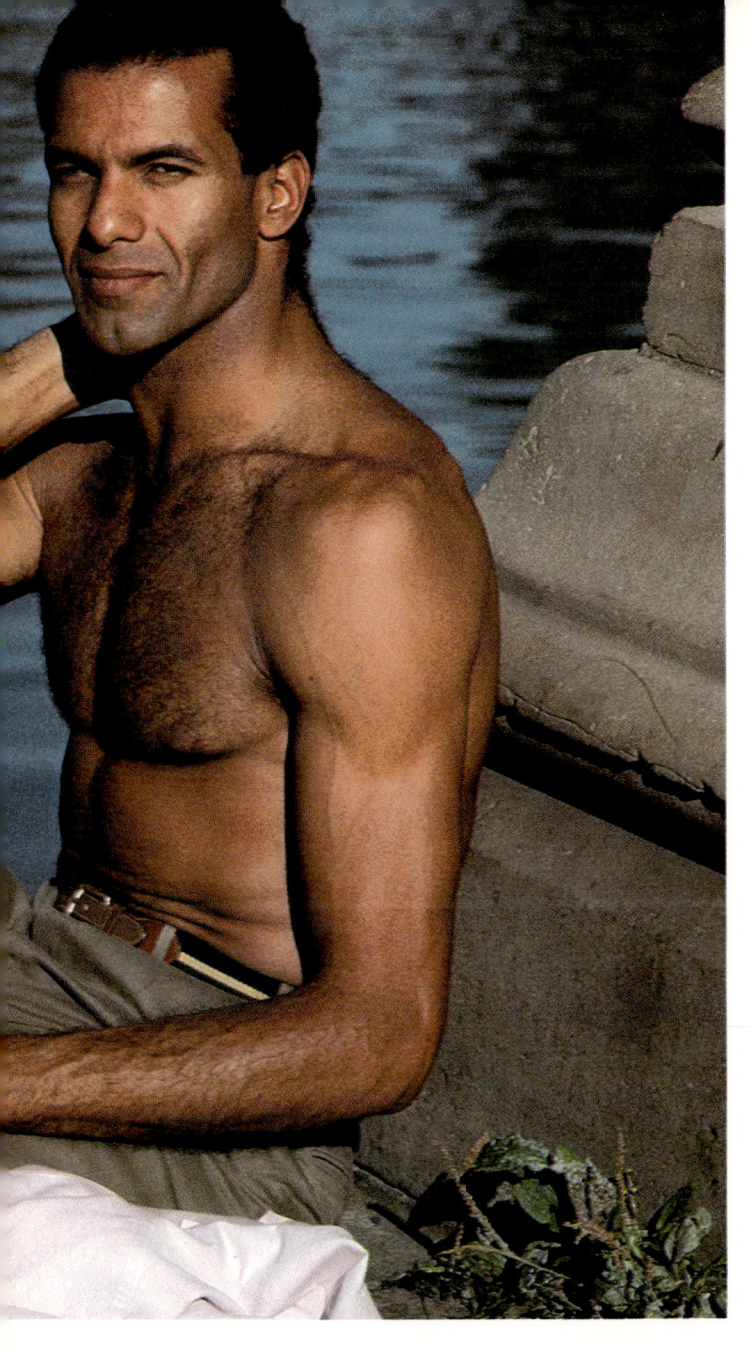

To facilitate his personal growth, Charles has embraced two interests. One is a special self-defense program that he has studied for nine years — and taught to others for six. He describes the instruction as completely unique. "It's not for everybody. It's about more than self-defense. It's about getting to know yourself again. You've got to find out who it is you're defending, and we do that through exercise and energy. We shake a person's whole foundation."

In April 1982, Charles took another major step. He became a disciple of the spiritual leader Bhagwan Shree Rajneesh. "It's not a religion," he emphasizes. "It's a way of living, a search for the ultimate goal, for reaching man's highest potential — enlightenment." Charles has also changed his name to Swami Bodhananda, which means "bliss and awareness." One of his leader's few requirements has revamped Bodhananda's fashion style: it is suggested that disciples wear red or orange clothes. How do people in the fashion business react to these changes? "Not always honestly," says Bodhananda. "Some people think I've gone crazy. But the ones who really know me think, if anything, I've gone sane."

Bodhananda

Vital & Not So Vital Statistics
Birthdate: June 21, 1949
Height: 6'2"
Weight: 180 lbs.
Hair: Brown
Eyes: Brown

Personal Favorites —
Designer: Jeffrey Banks
Movie: *The Empire Strikes Back*
Actors: Peter Finch; Dustin Hoffman
Actress: Goldie Hawn
Snack: Avocado and cheese sandwich
Drink: Vichy water
Vacation Spot: Barbados
Hobbies: Self-defense; tennis; roller skating
Agency: Elite, New York City

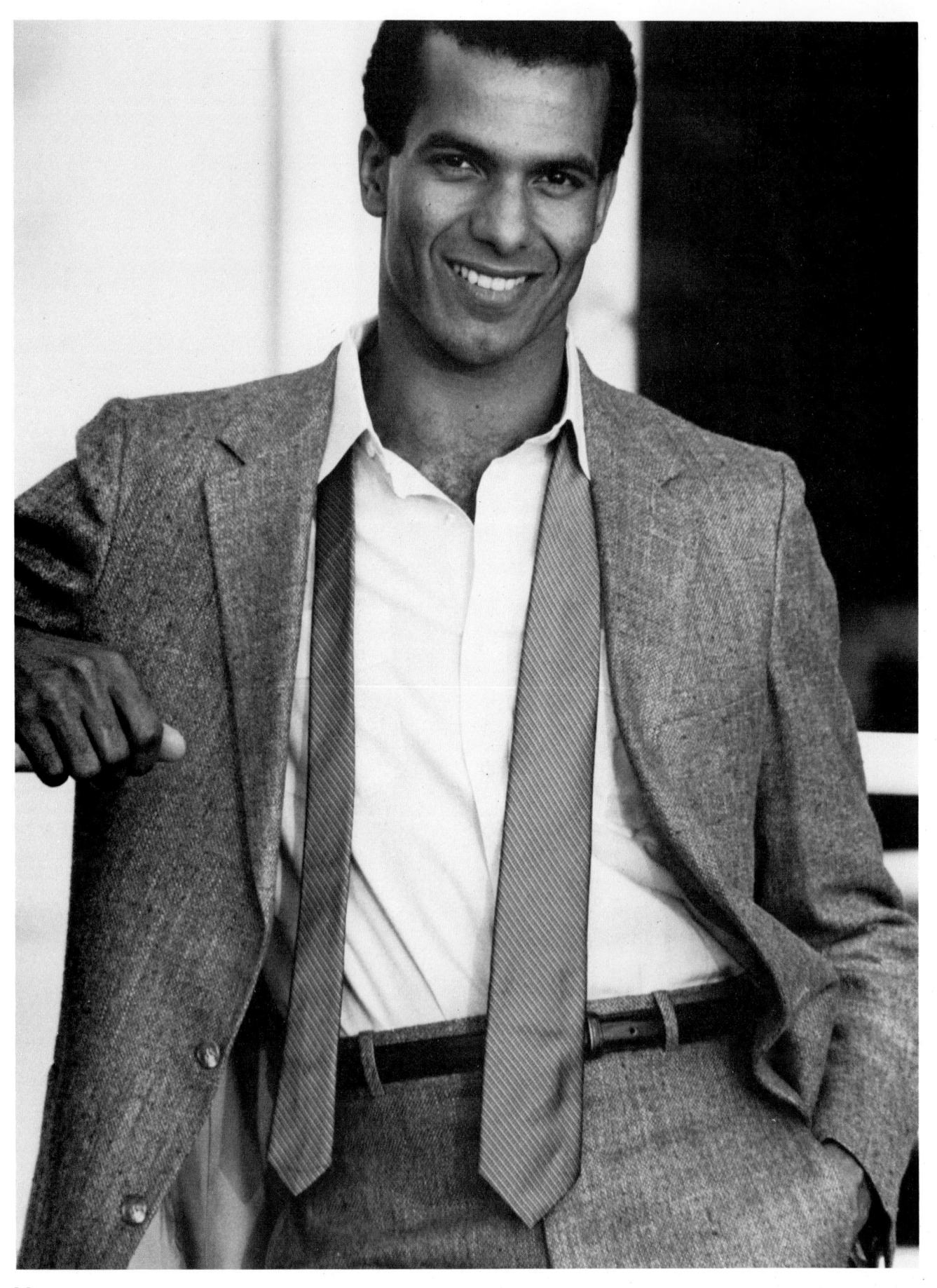

"
The black man is more
concerned about his dress outside
of his job.
He needs to present more of an image to get ahead.
If I dress nicely, people look upon me a
certain way. If I dress in my funky coat, they immediately get
a different impression.
"

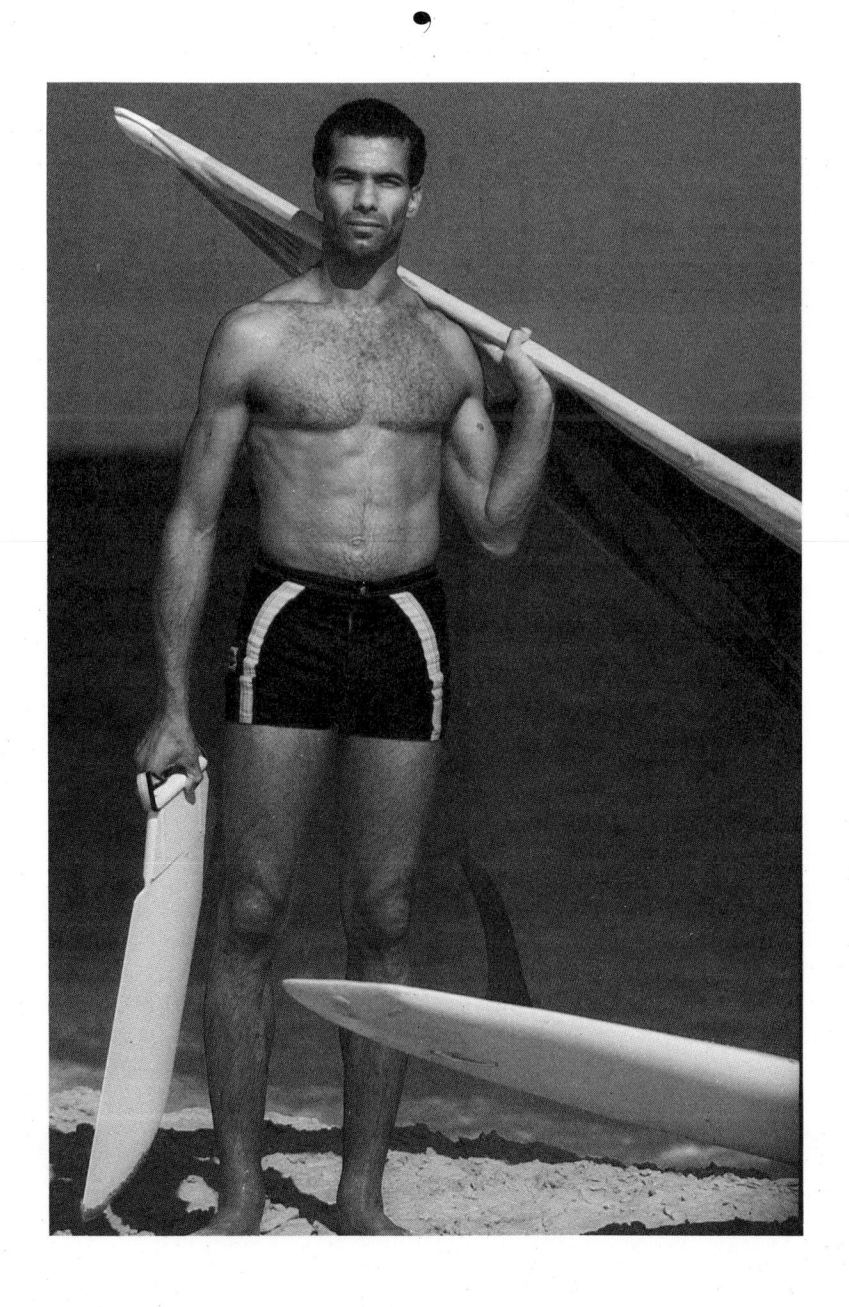

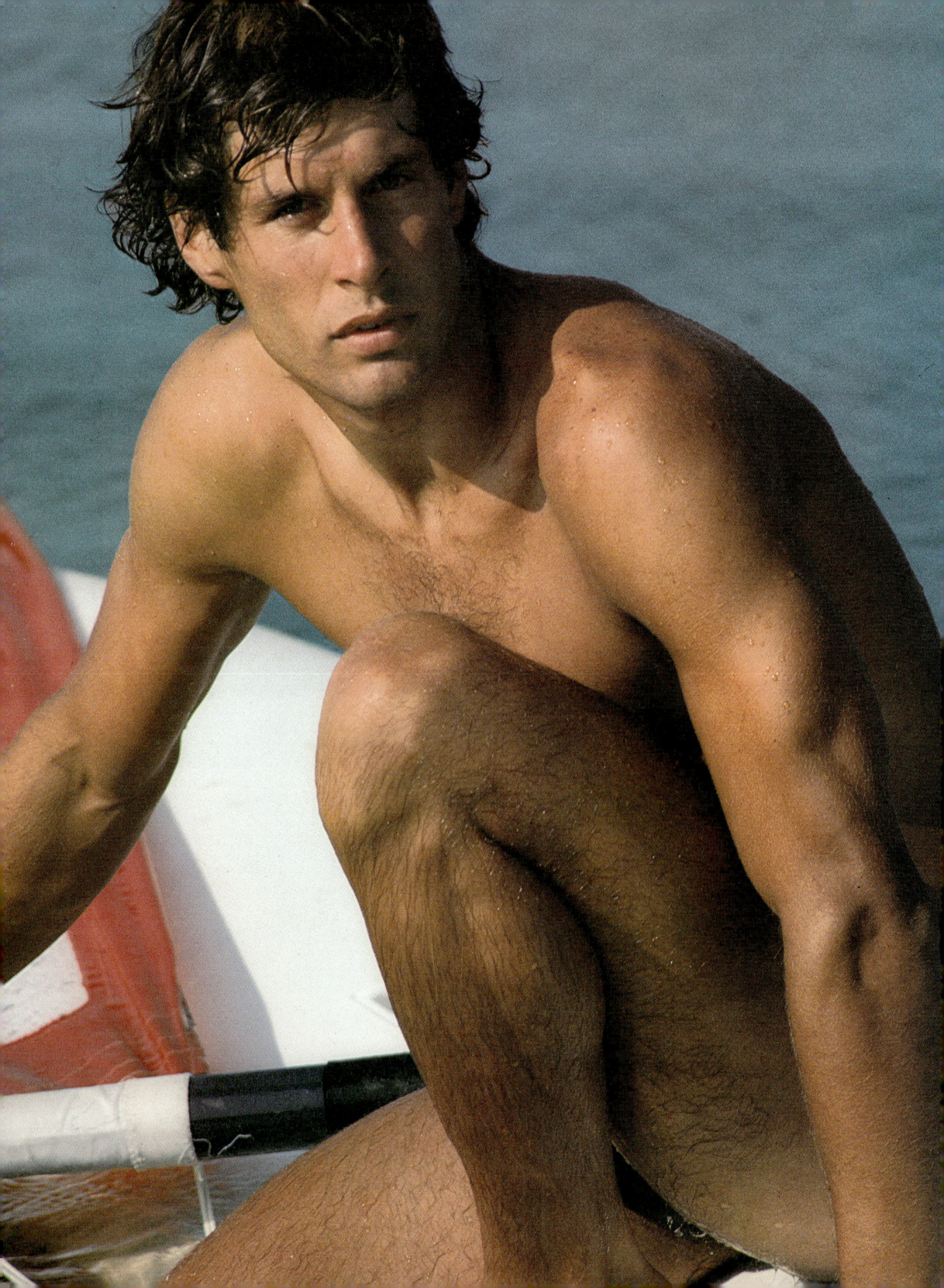

Jeff Aquilon

In his everyday faded jeans and T-shirt, Jeff Aquilon doesn't look much like a trailblazer — particularly a *fashion* trailblazer. But appearances are deceiving. Perhaps no model has done more to change the face (and body) of fashion in the 1980s than this California lifeguard who was discovered while still a water polo standout at Pepperdine University. When Bruce Weber first featured Jeff in a now-famous underwear spread in the *Soho Weekly News* in 1978, Aquilon became an overnight sensation, and male modeling underwent a revolutionary change. Gone was the high-fashion face that was all cheekbones. In its place, as personified by Jeff, was an American, athletic, healthy-looking virile man. Recalls Jeff, "When I first came to town and went out on interviews for jobs, people would say to me, 'God, this is so refreshing. You're not a New York model at all.' It was summer, and I'd ride my bike to appointments and wear shorts to interviews — and that was considered real different. The art director of GQ told me I couldn't wear shorts, that this was New York. I didn't want to offend anyone, but I didn't want to change either. Why should I have? I knew the reason I was here in the first place was because of who I was. Now, of course, everybody wears shorts and rides their bikes to interviews."

With his square jaw, swimmer's muscularity, and ingenuous smile, Jeff bridged the classic fashion type and the new American male. But, in his objective, down-to-earth manner, Jeff credits his superstardom in part to cultural changes. "I think I arrived in New York at just the right time," he observes. "The sixties and the seventies were about being crazy and doing all sorts of things to your body — *overdoing* things. But the eighties are about refinement and conditioning. You didn't see that in advertising before. When I got here, people were ready for a sense of somebody who looked

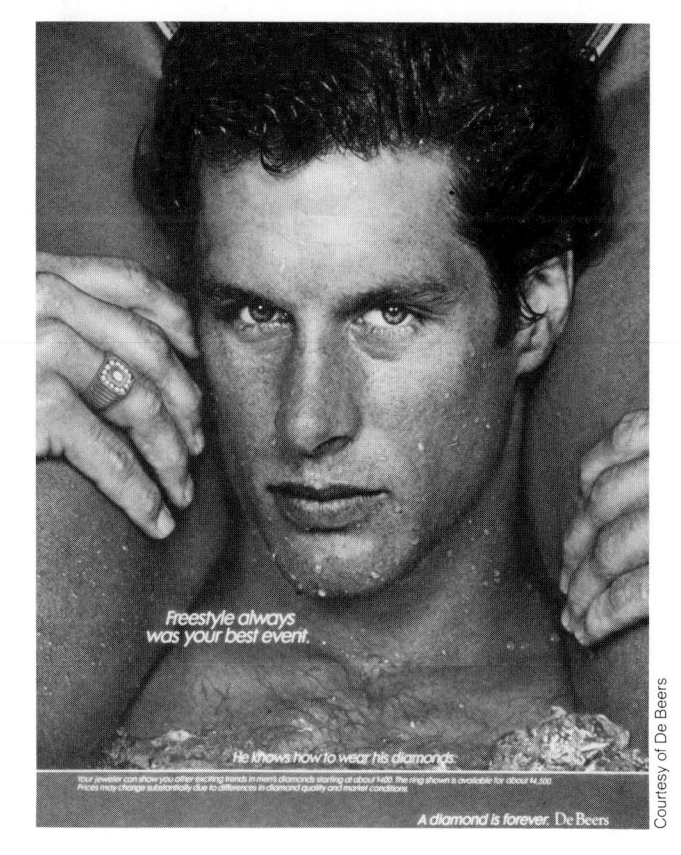

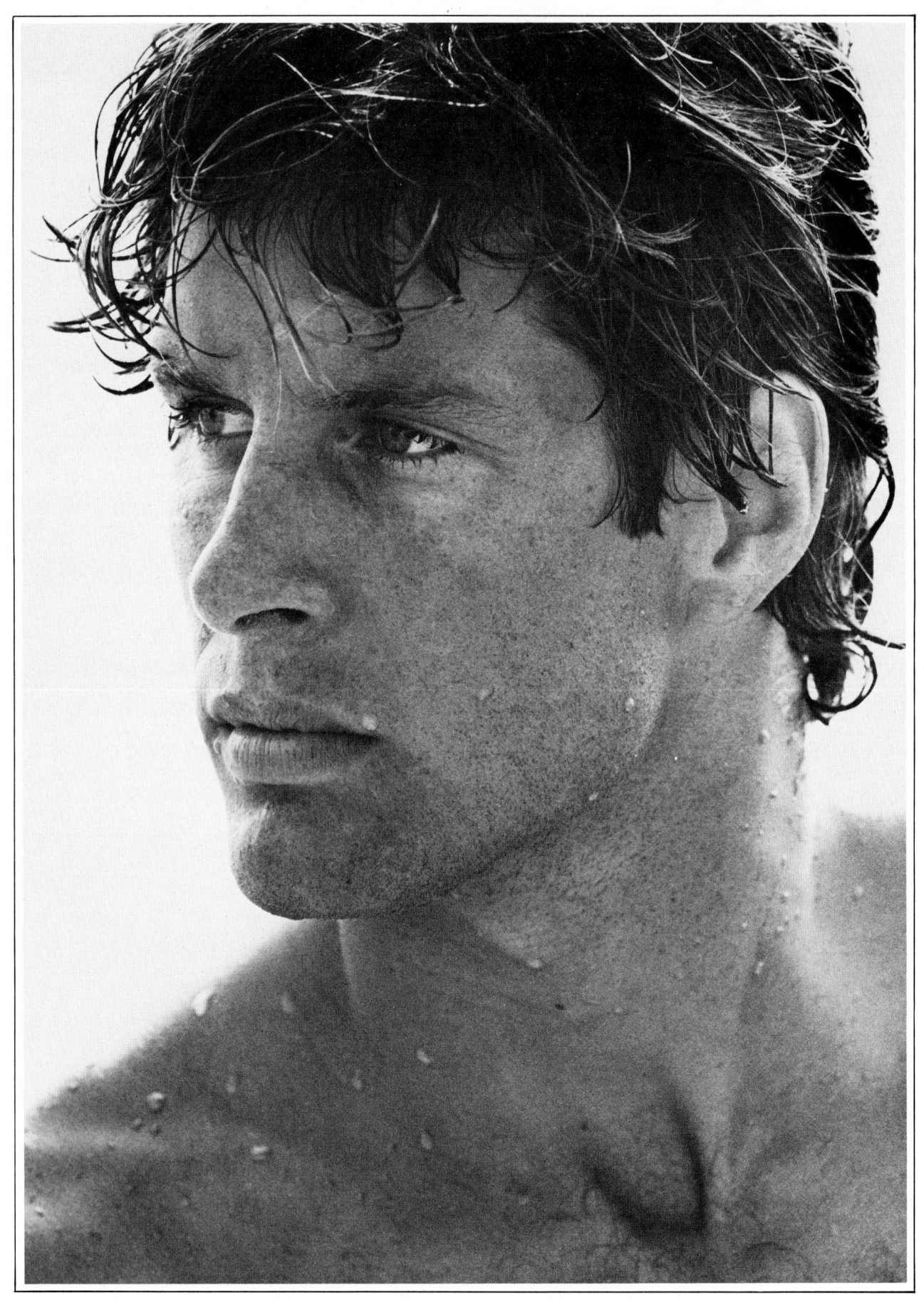

good, who looked healthy. It just *worked* for me. If I'd come here in the sixties, people would have laughed at me. I wouldn't have worked at all."

Jeff's athletic image began long before he ever got in front of a camera. He grew up in Santa Barbara, California, where "I spent any free time I could at the beach." Jeff recalls, "Any day the waves were up, I missed school to go surfing and got back to school in time for water polo practice." A 1979 graduate of Pepperdine with a degree in business administration, he attended college on full scholarship. Jeff was captain of the water polo team at Pepperdine, and was encouraged to consider modeling by several acquaintances, including the director of the Los Angeles Ballet. At first, Jeff balked. "I knew nothing about modeling," he says. "I thought the people in those pictures were just some producer's kids. I never looked at *GQ* or *Vogue*. I knew nothing about fashion. I wore a bathing suit, and that's all I worried about. I still hate the way clothes confine you." Spurred on by friends, Jeff signed with a California agency and began a halfhearted, part-time career as a model. "If I had done then what I really felt like doing, I would be a starving architect now," he says. "But I was getting out of college, and I didn't have anything better to do. I didn't want to take resumes around." Shortly thereafter, *GQ* came into town looking for new faces. Jeff's face was more than new; on the day of his *GQ* meeting, it was distinguished by two black eyes he'd suffered the night before in a water polo match. With those two black eyes, fashion history was rewritten, and Jeff's reputation as a rugged sort solidified.

In his pictures, Jeff is as much a strong, silent type as an athletic type. He has patented a frequently imitated sultry gaze known in the industry as the "your-dog-just-died" look. That distinctive expression has created as much a sensation as Jeff's athleticism. He explains, "When I first started, I wasn't really pouting. I was just expressionless. It was a gaze – no reaction to anything, like the way I looked over the water when I was lifeguarding." In actuality, Jeff considers himself more carefree than those pictures suggest. But he cautions that there's still an element of him in those moody photographs. "I don't do much acting," he says. "It's all *me*. When I do a picture, I'm thinking of something. Thoughts are going to determine how your eyes, face, everything is going to look. If you're thinking something intense, it'll come across in your face." Jeff acknowledges that circumstances sometimes affect his expression. For those legendary *Soho* shots, he says, "I flew in on the red-eye flight from California. I got here at six in the morning, went right to the studio and we shot until twelve. Coming in off the red-eye had some-

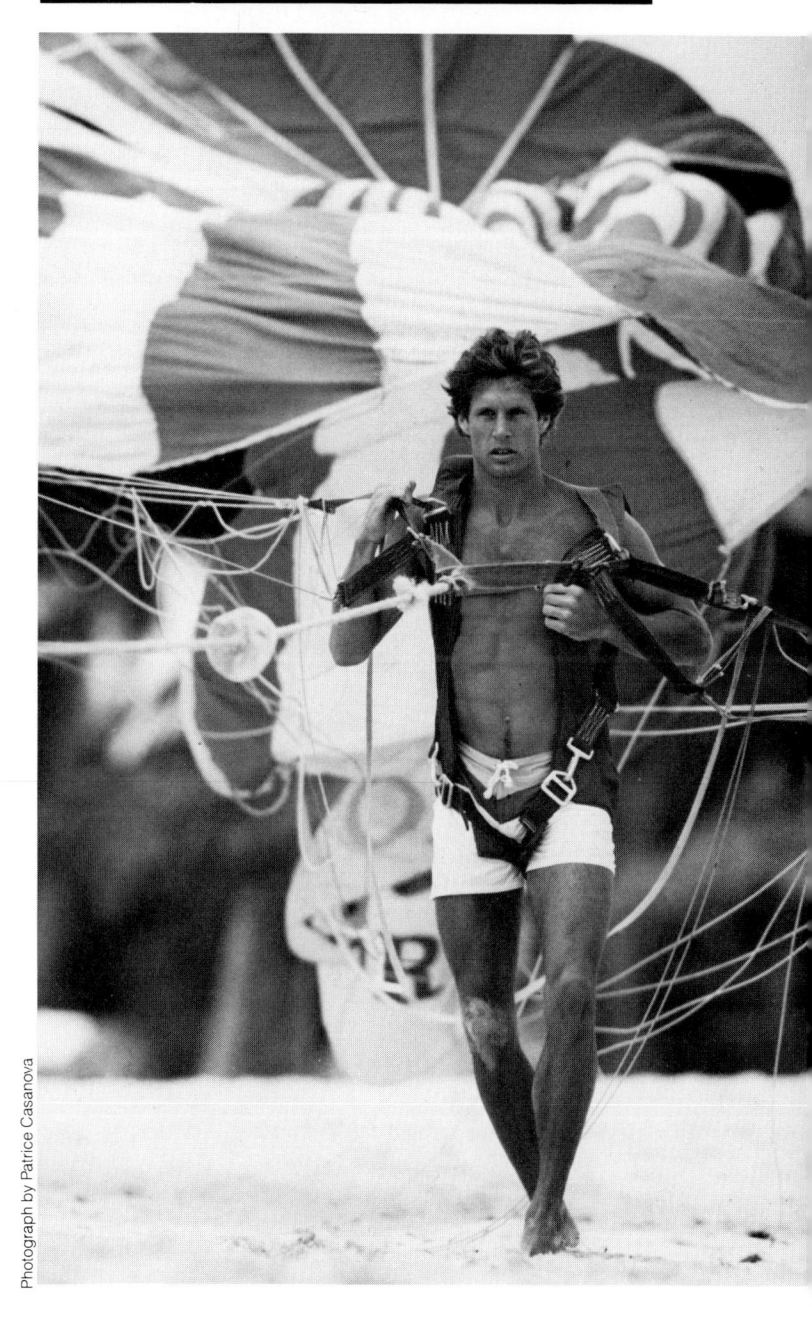

Photograph by Patrice Casanova

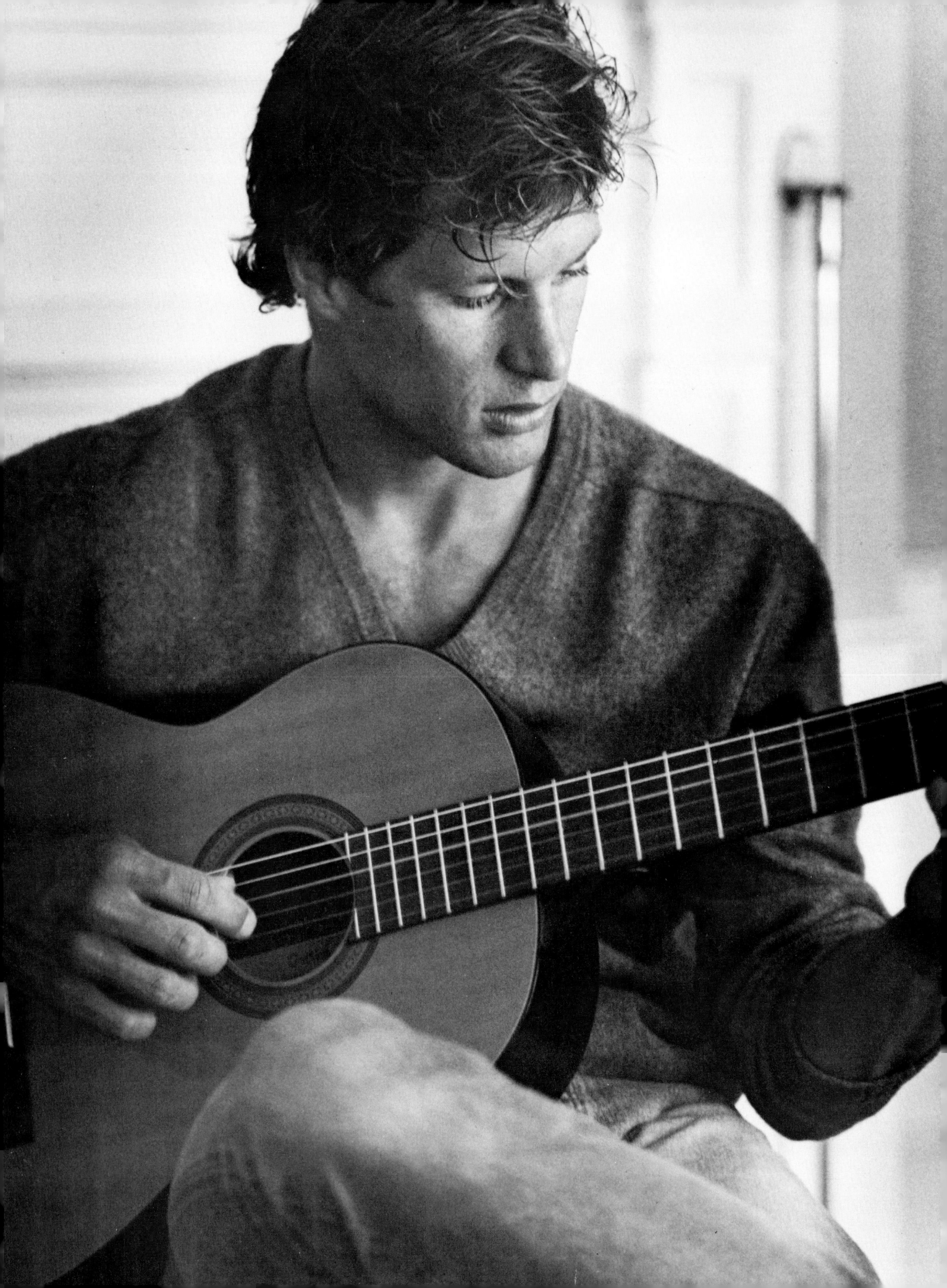

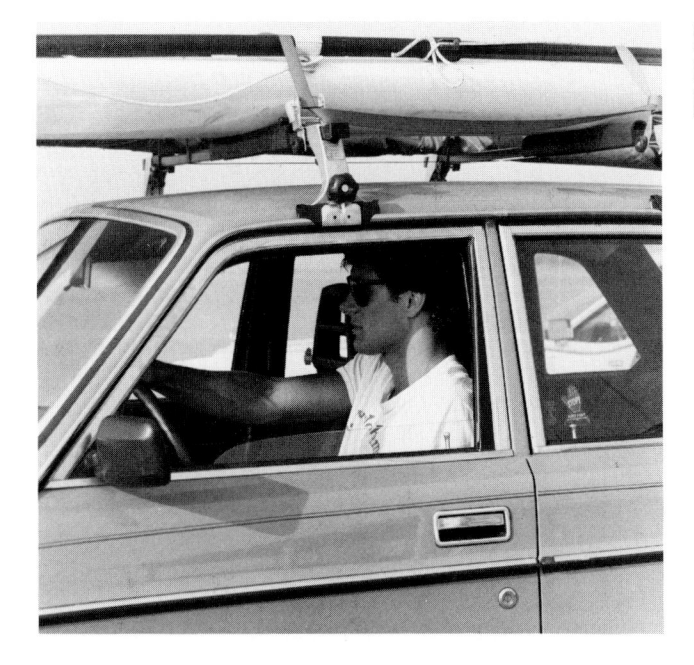

> People read things into pictures that I never would have thought of. But you can't worry about the reaction to pictures. In this business, you get every kind of reaction.

thing to do with that deranged look in my eyes."

You can take the beach kid out of California but you can't take the California kid out of Jeff Aquilon. His most frequent fashion statement is a pair of jeans, and he wears shorts well into October. Despite his superstar status, Jeff lives in a well-furnished but modest one-bedroom apartment on Manhattan's West Side. He and his wife, model Nancy Donahue Aquilon, also own a home in the town of Bellport, on Long Island. A two-model family, Jeff and Nancy have worked together on numerous occasions, but far-flung assignments frequently keep them apart. Jeff, for instance, may spend as much as six months a year traveling around the world on assignment. "Modeling is a pervasive part of our lives," he says. "The trouble is traveling, but there are lots of advantages. We really understand each other's lives and problems. We've got two great incomes. It'd be hard for me to be married to someone not in the business. It'd be hard to travel and do so many things and just have someone waiting at home for you all the time."

Jeff's pressure-cooker schedule prevents him from participating in many of his California pastimes. "I don't get to swim as much as I'd like," he says. "I ride my bike everywhere for exercise, and the rest of the time, I just grab what I can." He does not have a weight-training program, but he has developed a program for his prized Apple II computer. "I use it to keep track of this whole mess," he says. And he tries to spend what free time he can tinkering on his guitar. "I always wanted to play guitar. To me, it's a very restful, meditative, neat kind of thing. I should take lessons. But I don't have the time to look for a teacher, let alone take the lessons." Jeff would also like to return to what interests him most — his painting and drawing. "I've really only been able to think about watercoloring for the past three years. I would love to do too many things. That's my problem." Jeff studied business in college, but for the immediate future, all extra projects are on hold while Jeff retains his title as the industry's most sought after male model. "Modeling has taken up all my life for the last four years," says Jeff. "I'm not ready to fully pursue anything else. It would be futile to try. This is just too good."

Jeffrey A. Aquilon
Vital & Not So Vital Statistics
Birthdate: September 21, 1957
Height: 6'
Weight: 165 lbs.
Hair: Light brown
Eyes: Blue
Personal Favorites —
Time of Day: Early morning
Snack: Vanilla ice cream and strawberries
Drink: Carrot juice
Movie: *Women in Love*
Book: *The Thorn Birds*
Car: Silver diesel Volvo
Town: Santa Barbara, California
Hobbies: Drawing; surfing; water skiing; playing the guitar; programming a home computer
Clothing Style: Bathing suits — "I hate clothes."
Cereal: Shredded wheat
Fantasy: "Being stranded in a chalet in the Swiss Alps with my favorite girl"
Vacation Spots: Saint Moritz; Bermuda; snow skiing in Vail, Colorado
Agency: Ford, New York City

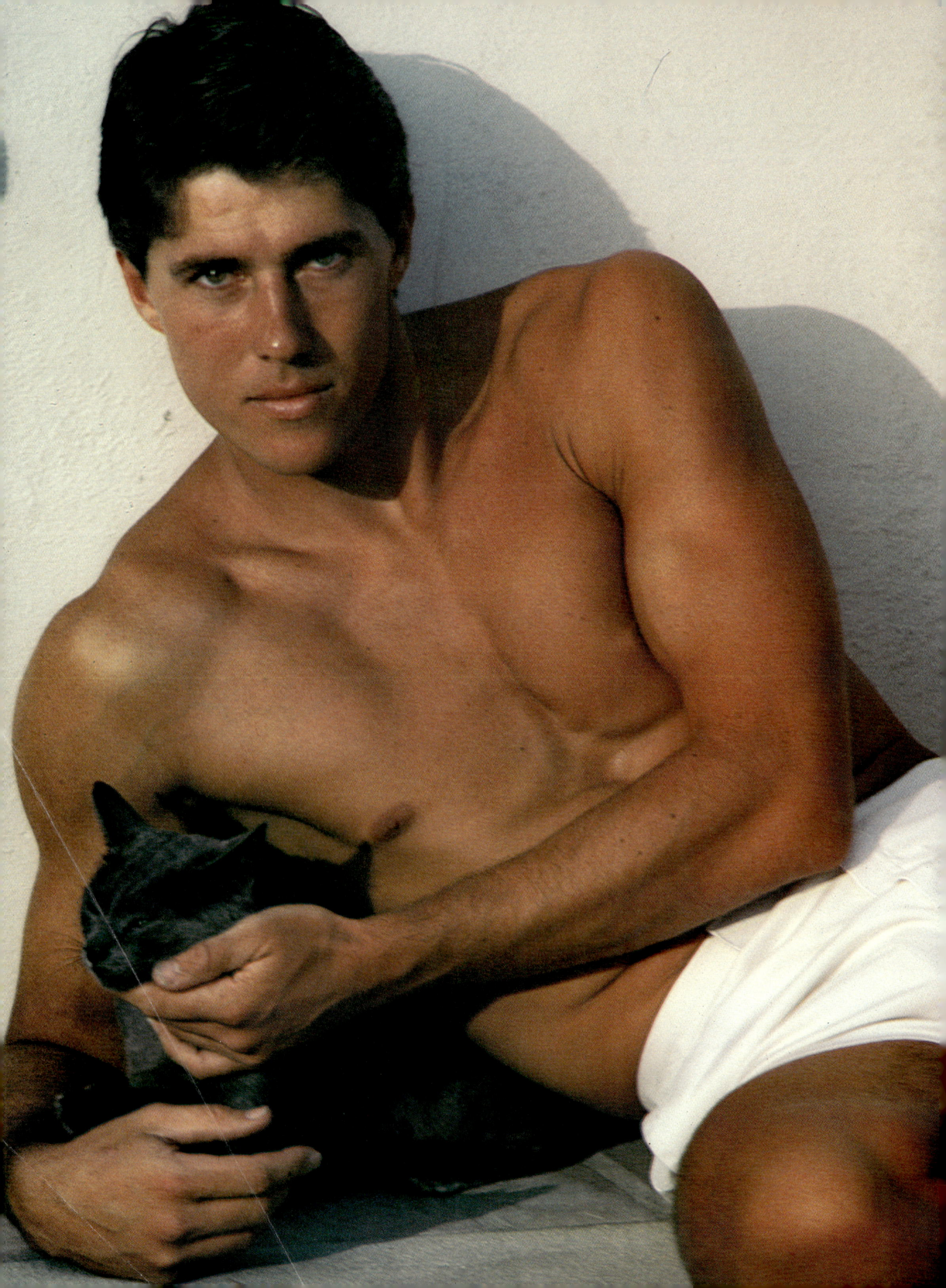

Tom Hintnaus

More often than not, Tom Hintnaus is up in the air. A national championship pole vaulter with an eye on the 1984 Olympic team, Tom regularly defies gravity and soars eighteen feet into the air. And if he's not soaring as the star of a high-powered track meet, he might be skiing over a jump or diving off a high cliff or hang gliding. Or possibly cruising in his ultra-light plane or bouncing toward the sky as he works out on his backyard trampoline. Tom doesn't particularly like having both feet on the ground: he's an eighties version of the daring young man on the flying trapeze. "I love the feeling of being up in the air," he says. "Things are just real clear up there. Maybe I was supposed to be a bird."

Maybe. Instead, Tom has unwittingly become a coast-to-coast sex symbol. As the statuesque model in Calvin Klein's controversial underwear advertisements, Tom is seen at bus stops and in magazines clad only in his shorts, leaning languorously against a white wall, framed by a stunning blue sky. Pictures of Tom's tanned, trim body, photographed to utmost advantage, are posted on office walls and bulletin boards. In fact, when the ad first appeared at New York bus stops, the photo became a black market prize. Despite the seeming anonymity of the shot, which was done with a low-angle lens that acentuates the shorts instead of the face, Tom doesn't mind the excitement the ad — and his body — have generated. "I've never stirred up so much attention in my life," he says. "But I feel removed from the controversy. I don't understand what all the commotion is about. It's just shorts. To me, it's like wearing Speedos when you swim. I didn't feel self-conscious doing the ad at all." The picture was shot by Bruce Weber on the Greek island of Santorini. "It's a photographer's paradise," says Tom, "because of the whitewashed buildings and the blue of the sky. I didn't really know it was an underwear ad

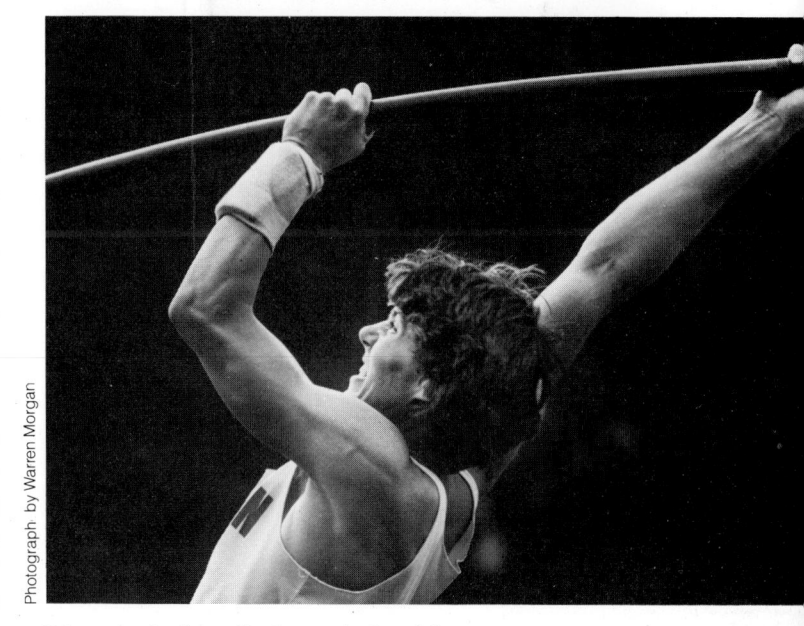

Photograph by Warren Morgan

"I love the feeling of being up in the air."

Calvin Klein Underwear

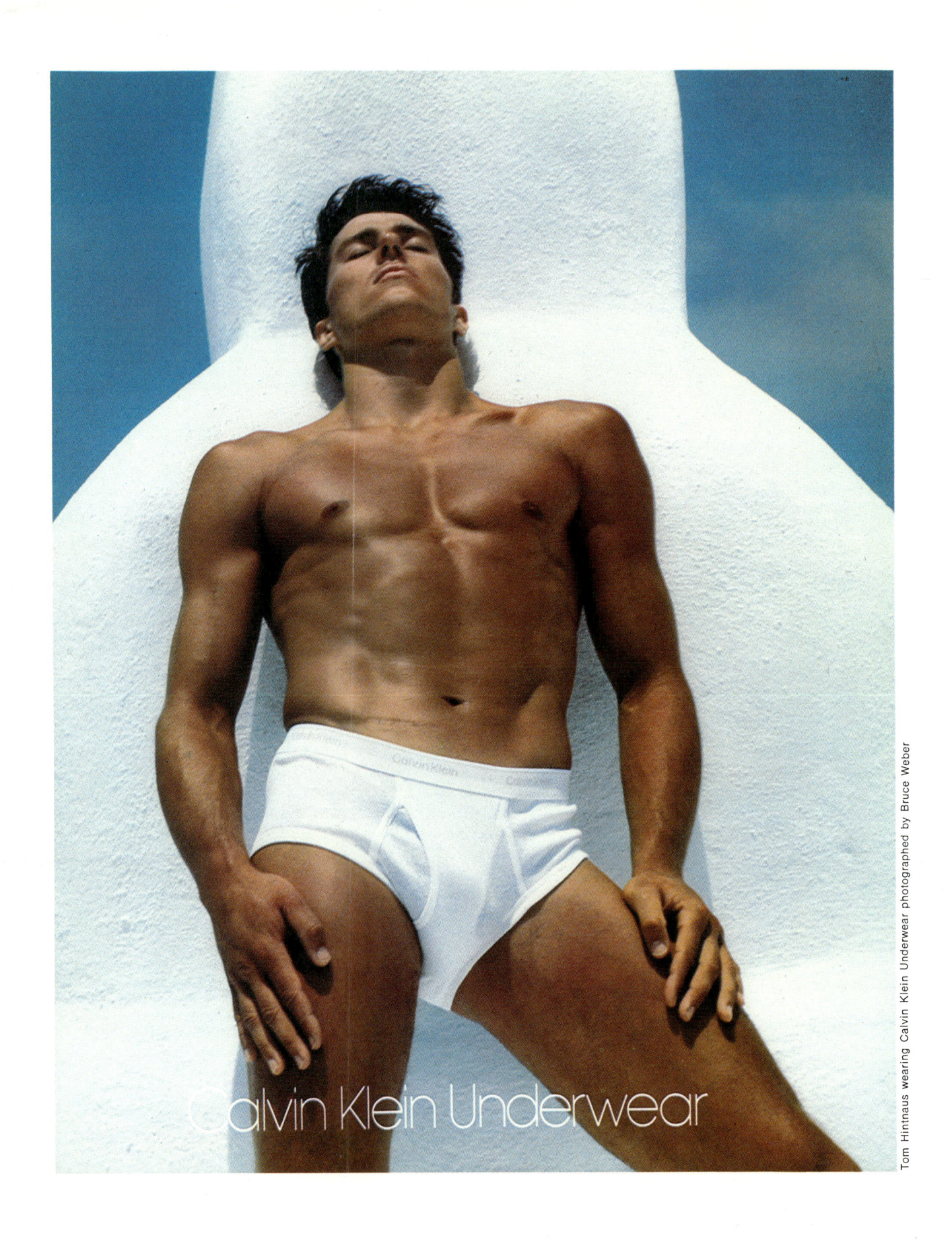

Tom Hintnaus wearing Calvin Klein Underwear photographed by Bruce Weber

until we got over there. But I knew if it was going to be Bruce Weber shooting, it would be classy stuff."

Until this attention-getting opportunity came his way, Tom expected that he would scale the ladder of fame and fortune by pole-vaulting. For several years, he's been recognized as one of the country's top vaulters. Tom developed his athletic talent at an early age. He first saw a pole-vaulting competition at the age of eight. "I said, that's what I want to do." He started to practice with a bamboo pole in the backyard, and he quickly climbed, so to speak, to the top. In high school, he won state and then national meets. In 1980, he placed first in the U.S. Olympic trials, but President Carter's boycott of the 1980 Summer Olympics in Moscow prevented Tom from a shot at international competition. Now, he's training intensely for the 1984 event.

"I love pole vaulting because it's all the sports rolled up into one," observes Tom. "You have to have speed, strength, coordination, air awareness, gymnastic skills. You have to use everything you have to get yourself over that pole. In a way, it's a dangerous event, and some people think I'm crazy, but there's a thrill when you're flying over the pole, and you get higher than you ever thought you could."

Tom was first approached about modeling when his wholesome looks and gymnast's frame caught the attention of David Eisenlohr, a part-time photographer for *Track and Field News,* during a 1979 meet. The photographer met Tom and related Jeff Aquilon's trek from water polo star at Pepperdine University to top fashion model in New York. Under the guidance of the photographer, who has since become his manager, Hintnaus began to build a portfolio and soon signed with the top agency in Los Angeles. For Tom, modeling is an adventure as well as a sensible way to finance his pole-vaulting training. "If I had to work a nine-to-five job every day, it would end my pole-vaulting career right away," he says. "This gives me plenty of time for practice." In fact, Tom has only one small complaint about modeling. "In the pictures," he says, "you have to look different, you have to look like you mean business, be serious. Away from the camera, I'm always smiling and laughing and goofing around. So people who know me don't recognize me in magazines."

Although his looks are quintessentially American, Tom was in fact born in Brazil. His parents are former Czechoslovakian citizens who escaped from their homeland in 1948. When they wanted to move from Germany to the United States two years later, they could only get clearance for Brazil, and consequently moved there. When he was two, Tom's family moved to California, where his father is an electronics company manager and his mother is an IBM inspector. Tom attended the University of Oregon with a major in telecommunications, and is preparing for the Olympics from his Manhattan Beach, California, home.

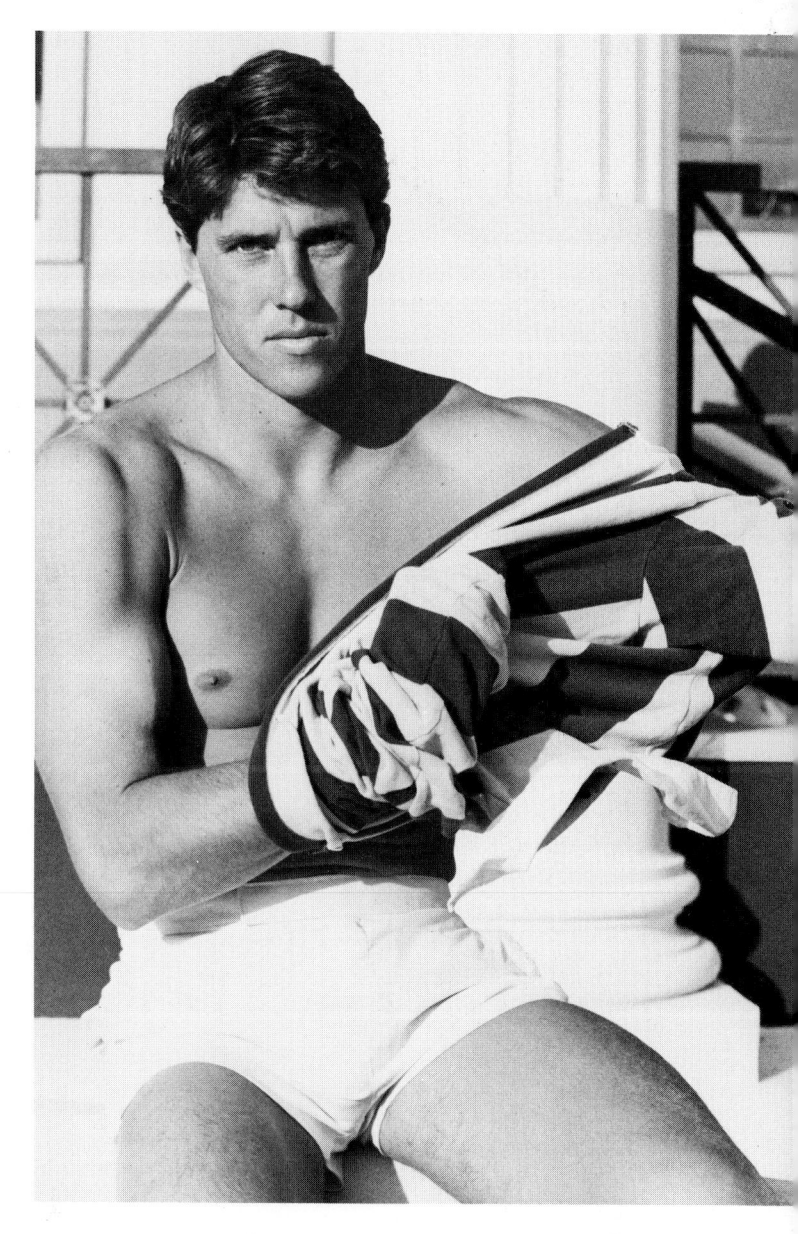

When Tom stops vaulting, he sees as his next hurdle a career in acting or stunt work. He's already appeared in the feature film *Can't Stop the Music,* and, for an NBC sports program, he has performed one news-making stunt: he vaulted onto the Great Wall of China. But all future goals are secondary to the fulfillment of his lifelong ambition: to perform well in the 1984 Olympics. "My whole energy is going into making the team," says Tom. "All my life, that's been my goal, and I've spent ten years training for it. It was taken away from me in 1980, but I'm going to give it my best shot for 1984."

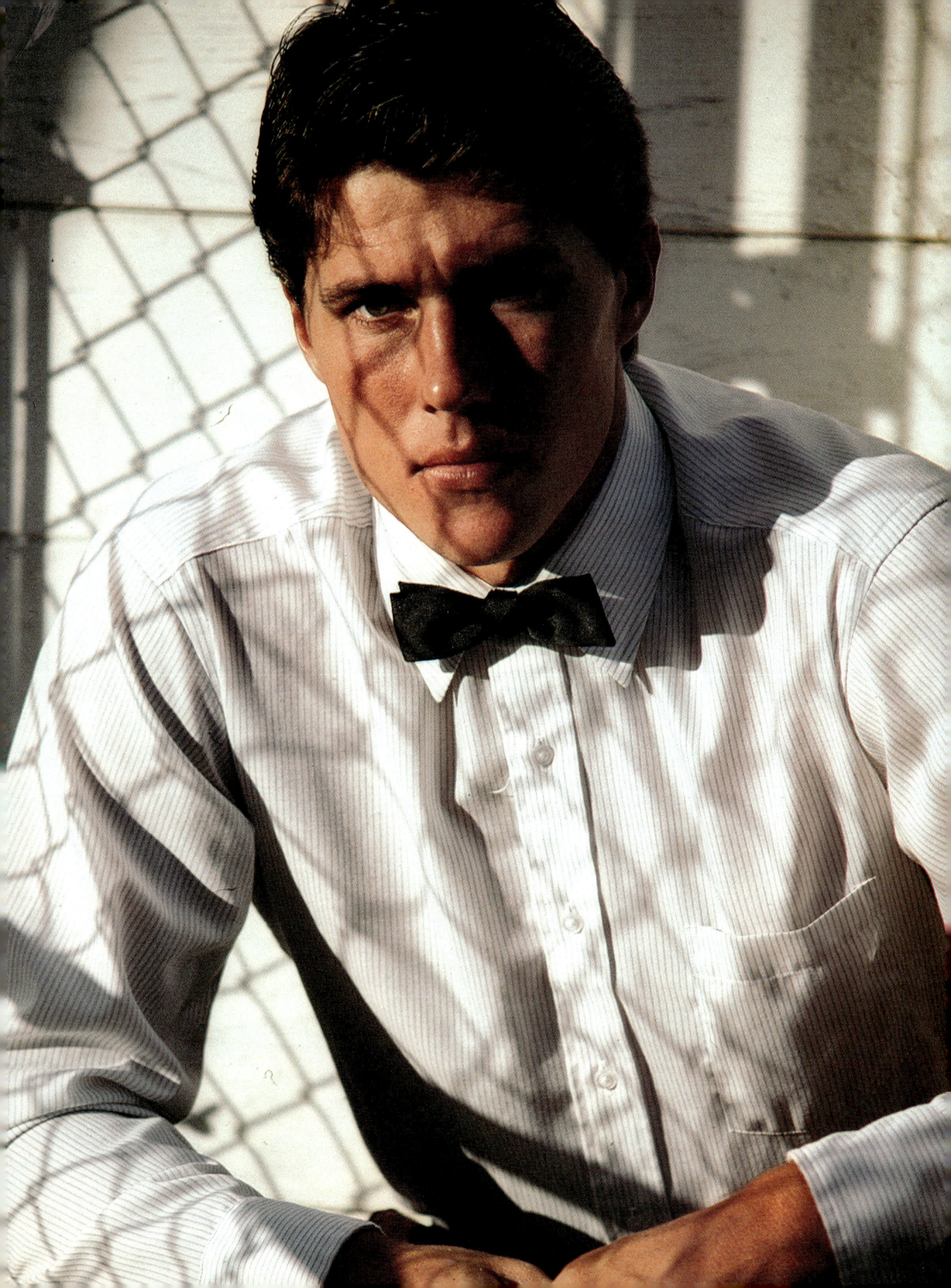

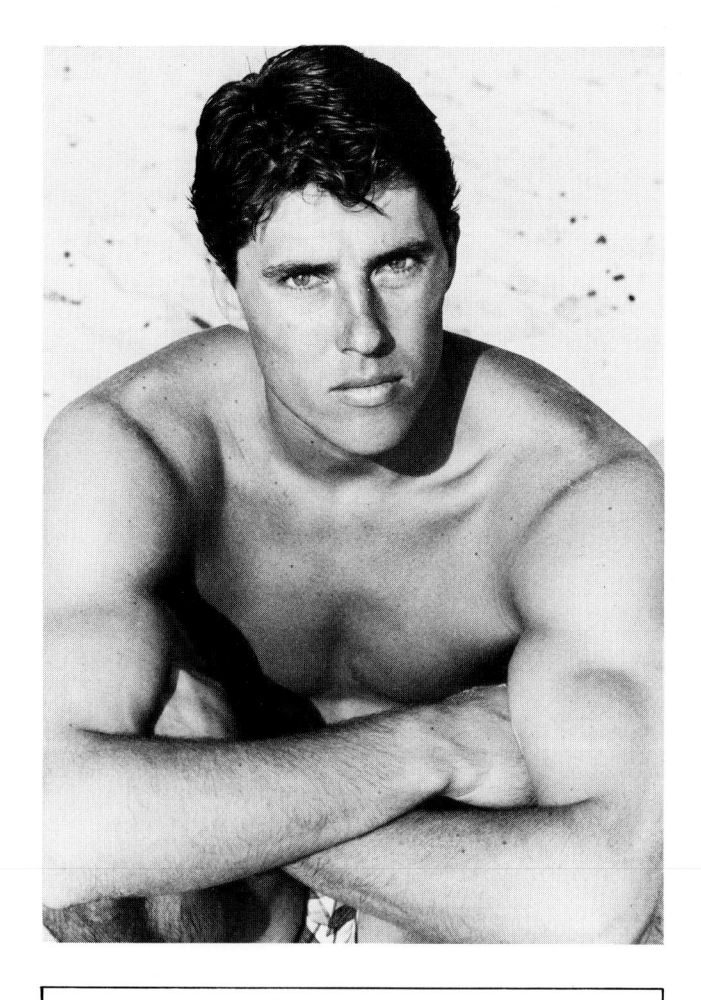

Some of my friends have given me a lot of hassle about being in my underwear. But I like the attention. Attention is attention.

Tom Hintnaus
Vital & Not So Vital Statistics
Birthdate: February 15, 1958
Height: 6′
Weight: 178 lbs.
Hair: Brown
Eyes: Green
Personal Favorites —
Town: Manhattan Beach, California
Vacation Spot: Hawaii
Drinks: Strawberry margaritas; Gatorade
Food: Pizza
Actors: Paul Newman; Cary Grant
Movies: *Raiders of the Lost Ark; Rocky III*
Hobbies: Surfing; skiing; hang gliding; ultra-light flying; woodworking
Color: Blue
Hangout: Tequila Willie's, Manhattan Beach
Dress Style: Casual — shorts
Music: Rock
Designer for Men: Calvin Klein
Cologne: Polo
Time of Day: Afternoon
TV Shows: *Dynasty; Hill Street Blues*
Ambition: "To make the 1984 Olympics, win the pole-vaulting Gold, and go on to '88."
Agency: Mary Webb Davis, Los Angeles

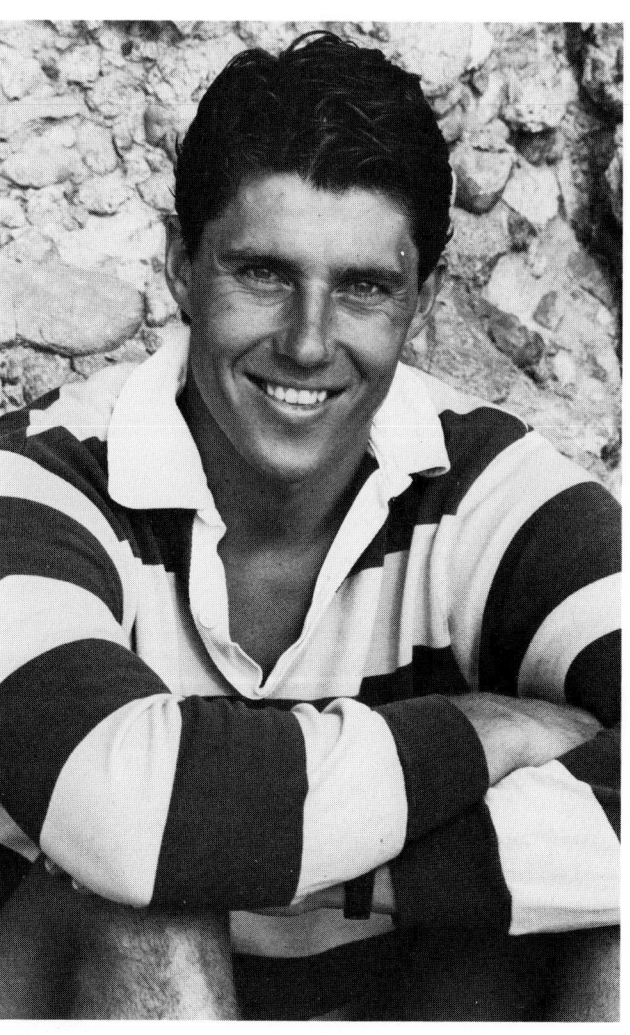

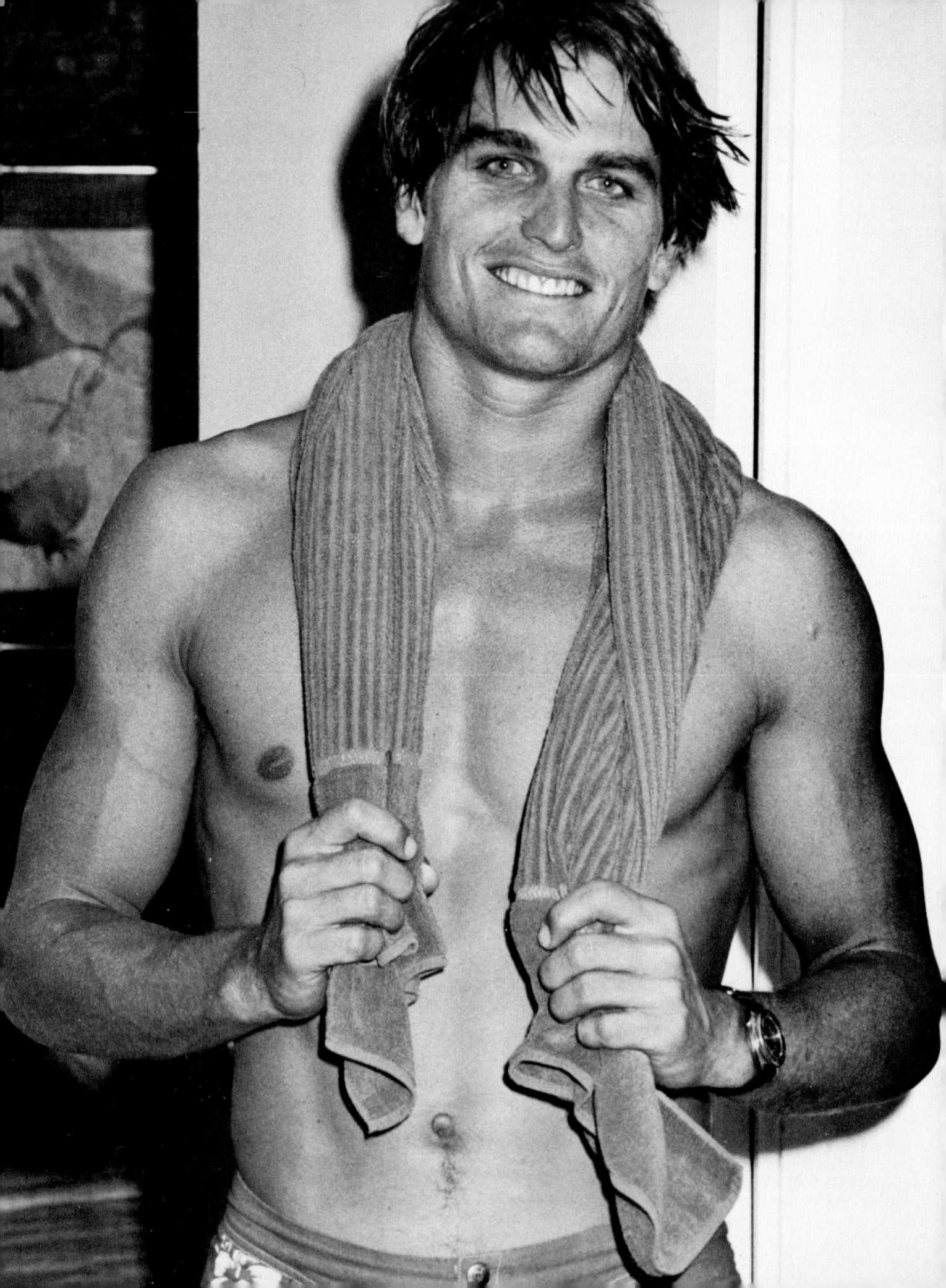

Buzzy Kerbox

Blond, blue-eyed, and perpetually wind-blown, Buzzy Kerbox looks as though he belongs on top of a wave – and that's just where Buzzy likes to be. A champion surfer based in Hawaii, Buzzy has traveled five times around the world in pursuit of the perfect wave. He's a bronzed believer in that legendary phenomenon known as the endless summer. And in his sunbleached way, Buzzy epitomizes another, very different phenomenon: the trend toward "model" athletes in fashion.

The Kailua Kid, as Buzzy is known on the surfing circuit, has a 1978 World Cup surfing title, his own surfboard label, and has suffered stitches in his head "probably ten times," estimates Buzzy. "Well, let's see," he says, totting up his injuries in the line of duty, "I've broken my nose, chipped my teeth, and once, during a contest, the nose of this guy's board was coming right for my vital parts. I covered them with my hand, but I ended up with stitches in my hand." Some models look rugged. Buzzy Kerbox *is* rugged.

In fact, Buzzy was in an Australian hospital recovering from a freak surfing accident when the subject of modeling was first raised. From the hospital, Buzzy phoned his parents in Hawaii to tell them about his condition. Instead, they told him that a photographer from the East Coast had called for Buzzy. While Buzzy had been flying through the breakers off Australia, Bruce Weber had been flipping through a surfing magazine in New York on the lookout for new, outdoorsy faces. Buzzy's sturdy looks and infectious smile caught his attention. After speaking to his parents, Buzzy called Bruce. Recalls Buzzy, "Bruce said, 'I'd like you to come to New York and do this shoot for *Vogue* magazine.' I just about fell over. He'd seen a 9"x3" picture of me with a surfboard and had convinced *Vogue* to use me."

Despite his weathered looks and way around a

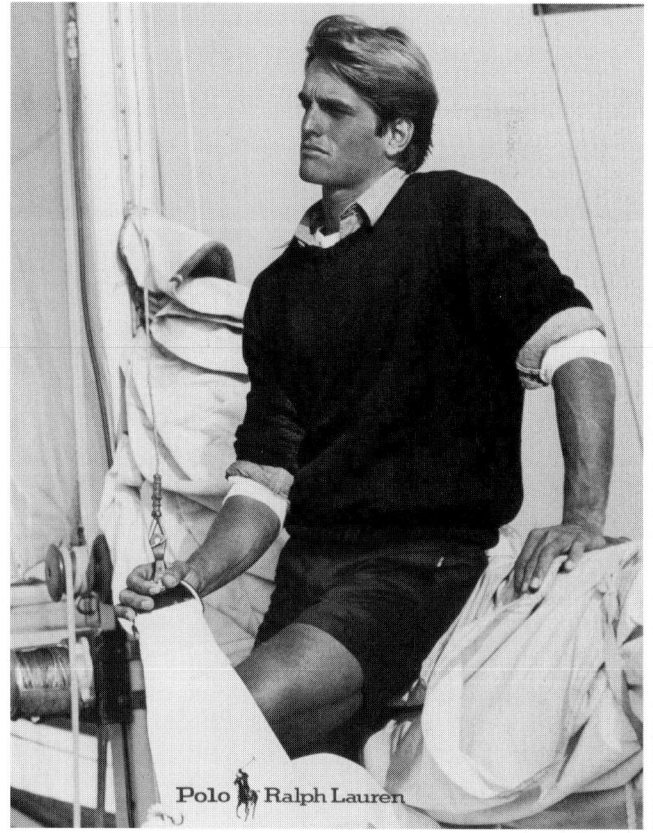

Polo by Ralph Lauren advertisement, photo by Bruce Weber

wave, Buzzy wasn't a born surfer. In fact, he spent his formative years landlocked on the mainland. Born and raised in Indiana, Buzzy was nine when his family moved to Hawaii. As a sportswriter once observed, "For Buzzy, life really began at age nine." Mr. Kerbox bought his son a surfboard and encouraged him to develop his talent. But Buzzy was considered an outsider in the close-knit world of amateur surfing on Oahu. He may be the Kailua Kid now, but he was the boy from Indiana then. At age seventeen, Buzzy surfed in his first professional event — and encountered twenty-five-foot waves. "They looked like they could kill you at any moment, and I was scared." After that, Buzzy divided his time between the beach and Windward Community College. During his first season on the pro circuit, he wasn't much noticed, and when Buzzy got any attention at all, it was for being the underdog. But Buzzy demolished that image with his upset triumph in the 1978 World Cup. "It had been my goal for so long," he says. "I never wanted to win every contest. There were just a few certain contests I wanted to win — to prove that I could to myself and to my father, who was always pushing me to win one. When I won the World Cup, I was famous for a little while. I had money for a little while." But Buzzy thinks he can be *too* laid back at times. He took a year off after his victory. "I didn't do anything in 1979," he says. "After a year, everything wore off. I was back to square one." For his comeback, Buzzy went Down Under and placed first in a 1980 Australian contest, taking home twenty thousand dollars.

As the quintessential beach boy, Buzzy finds his position in fashion awesome. And a bit bewildering. When he first saw his likeness on a huge billboard in New York's Times Square, he was stunned — and beamed with satisfaction. "It's a totally different world," says Buzzy, who sounds as star-struck with the fashion business as it is with him. "Having people fussing over my clothes and combing my hair. So different. But I'm pretty easygoing, and I get along with everybody, so it's fun." The fashion world sometimes bewilders his family too. Buzzy recalls, "For one shot, I had to rub dirt into a four-hundred-dollar shirt. My mom saw the photo and said, 'It's a great picture, but do you think you could wear a clean shirt next time?'"

Since entering the modeling business, Buzzy himself has been bitten by the shutterbug. Now, when a photographer isn't taking pictures of him, Buzzy is busy taking pictures of everything going on around him. "I love photography," he says. "I take stills and movies of whatever I'm doing: surfing or modeling. Some of the other guys have been around the world five times and never taken a single picture. I can look back on my pictures and remember the experience."

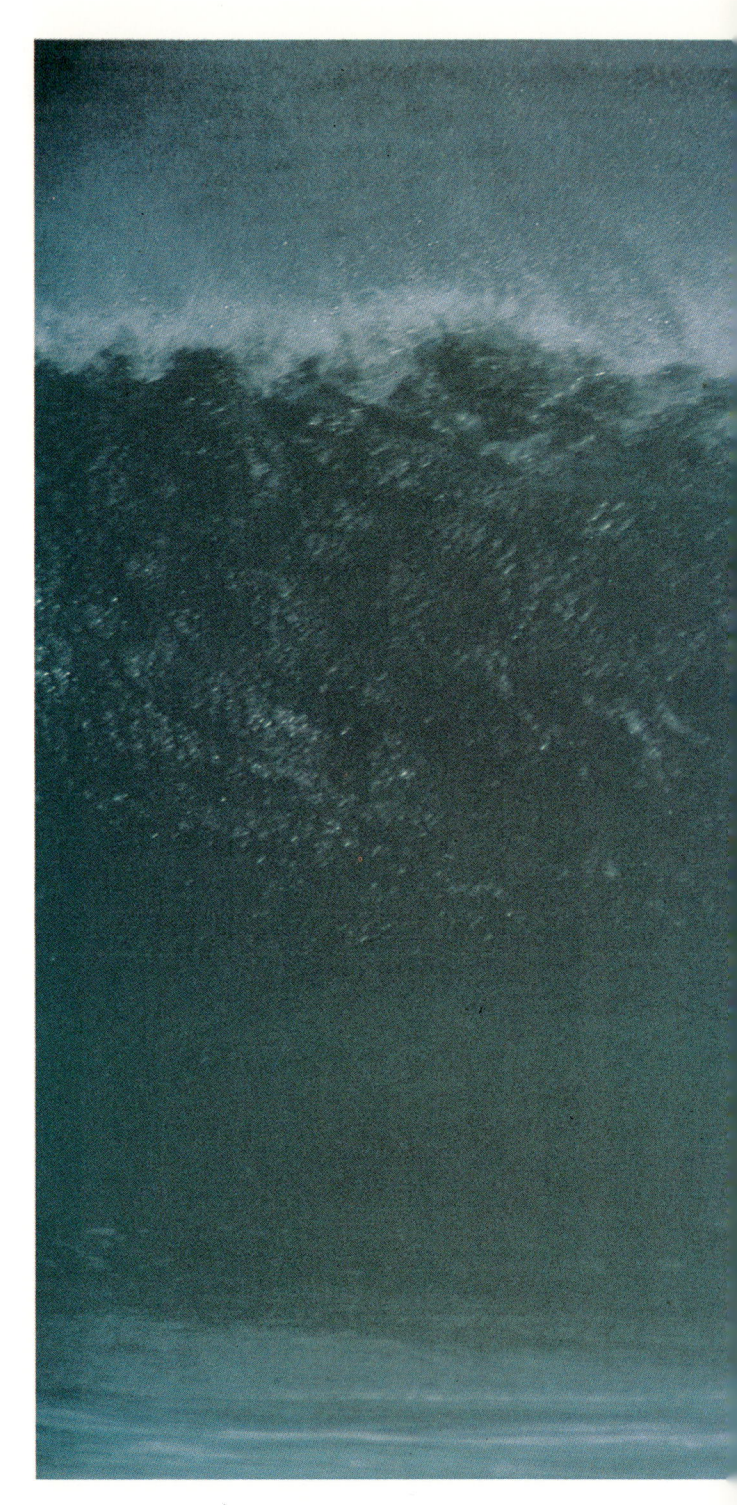

In his first *Vogue* spread with Bruce Weber, Buzzy happened to be wearing Ralph Lauren clothes. The designer saw the pictures, admired Buzzy, and put him under an exclusive contract — a rare and lucrative deal for a male model. Buzzy explains, "At one point, the Lauren people wanted

Photograph by Douglas W. Avery

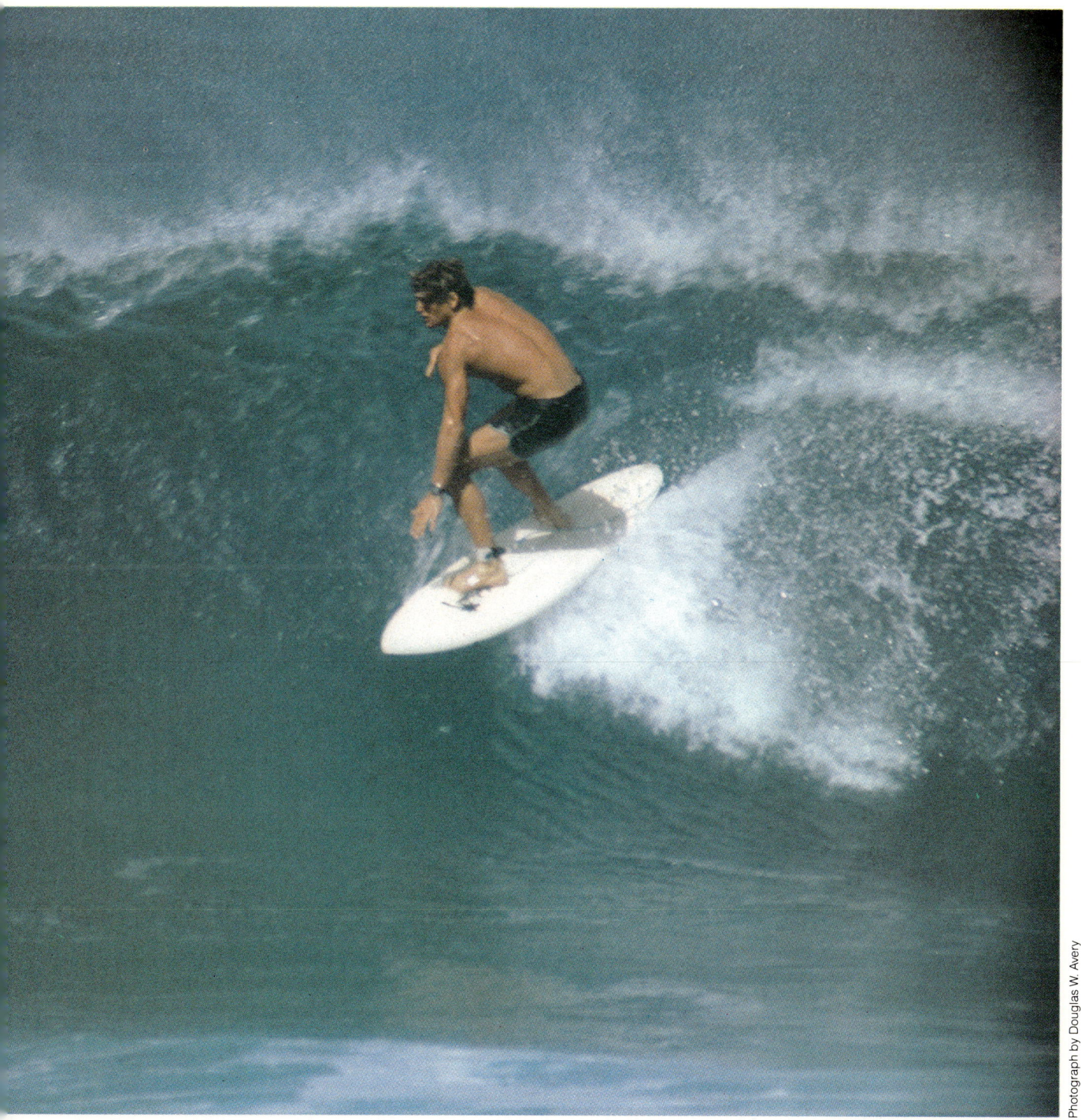

to do a shooting, and I couldn't because the World Cup was going on at the same time. After that, they decided to put me under exclusive contract so that I'd be available whenever they wanted. They made me an offer I couldn't refuse."

Buzzy currently spends six months a year at his home in Hawaii and six months traveling. "I'm in Hawaii three months at a time — when the surf is good on the North Shore." He ultimately wants to start an ocean-oriented enterprise that will enable him to incorporate his love for the water into his business life. But Buzzy isn't sure he can reconcile his fun-loving nature with the necessary bottom-line sensibility. He's not certain a beach boy can transform himself into a businessman. "I gotta admit I'm not a sharp businessman," observed Buzzy once. "I'm the kind of guy who ends up giving all his T-shirts away to friends."

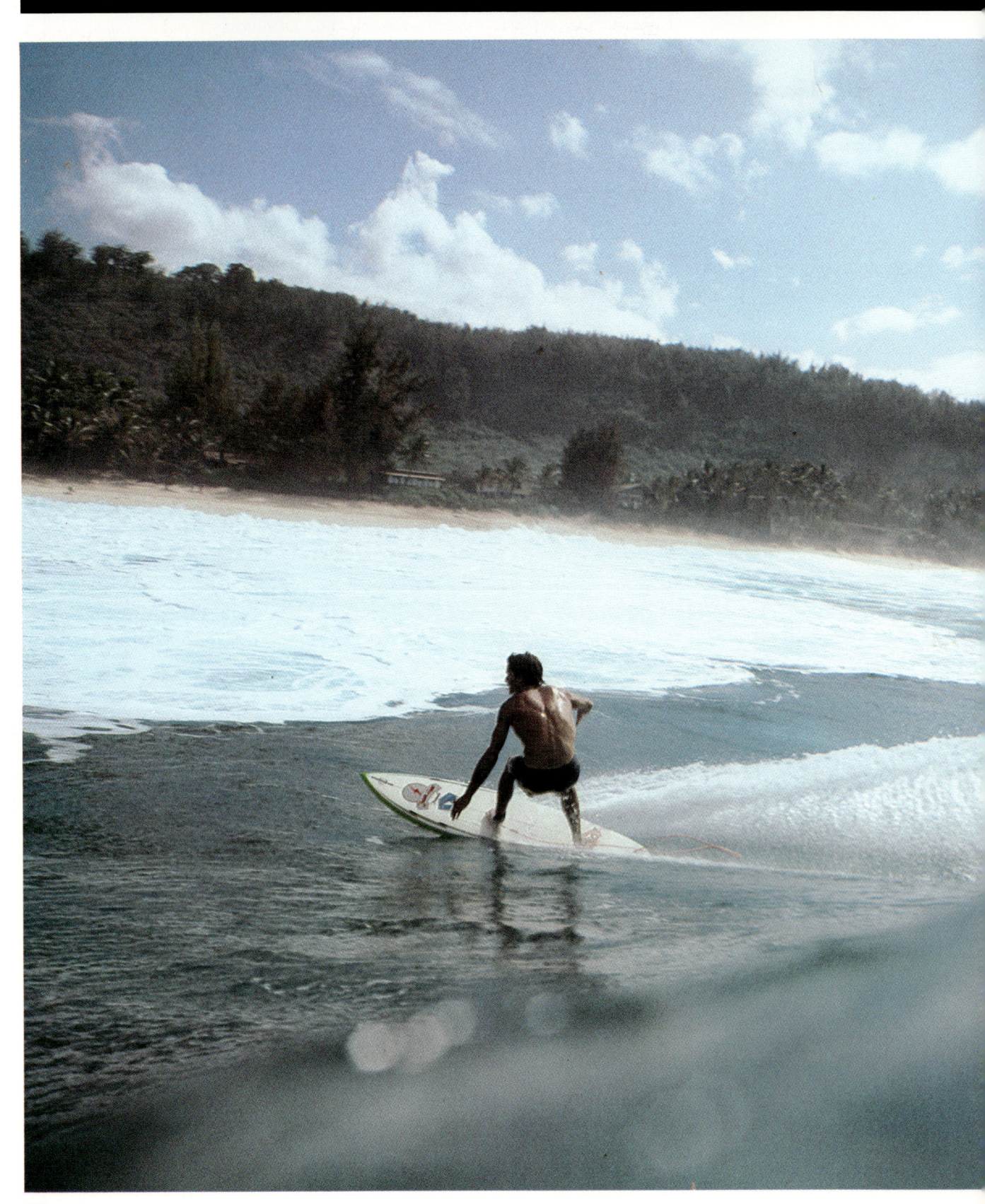

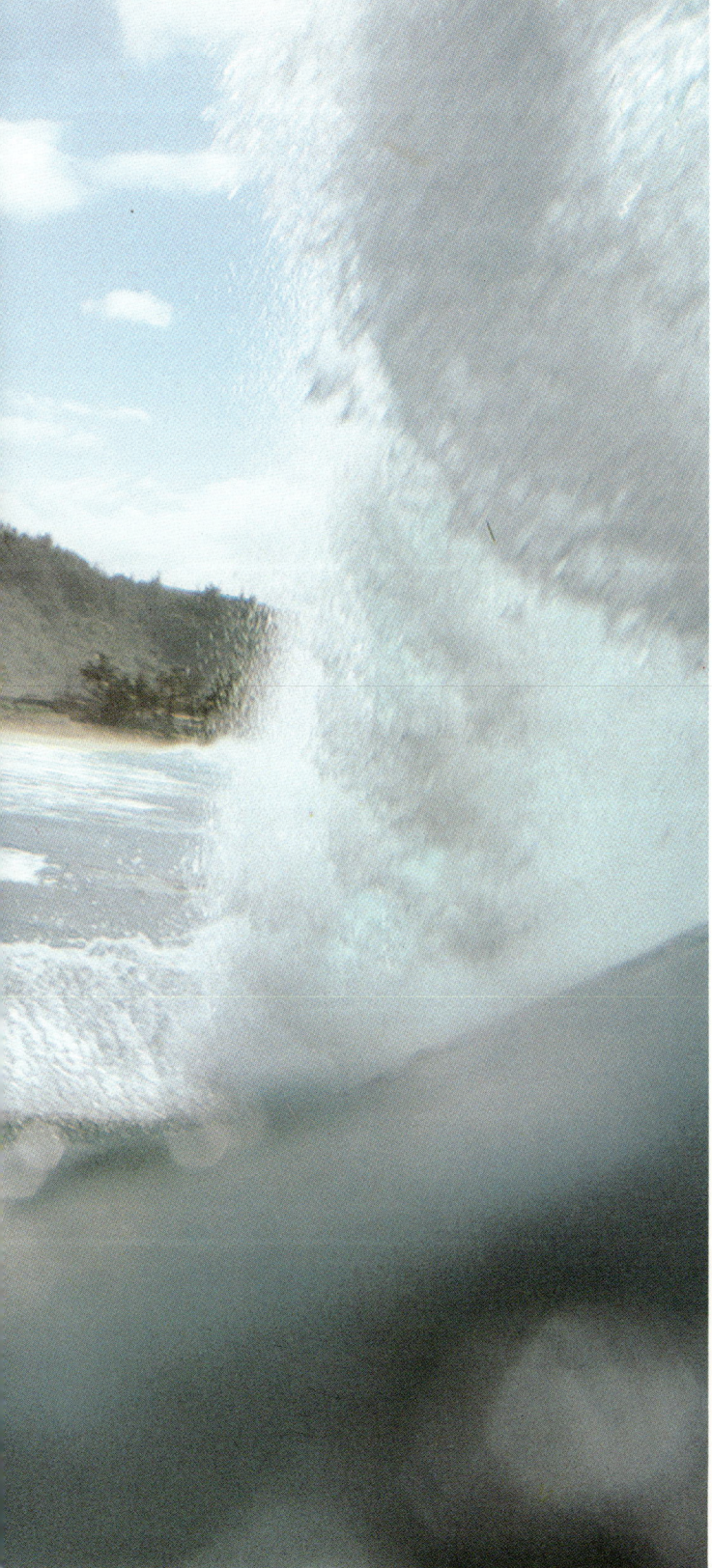

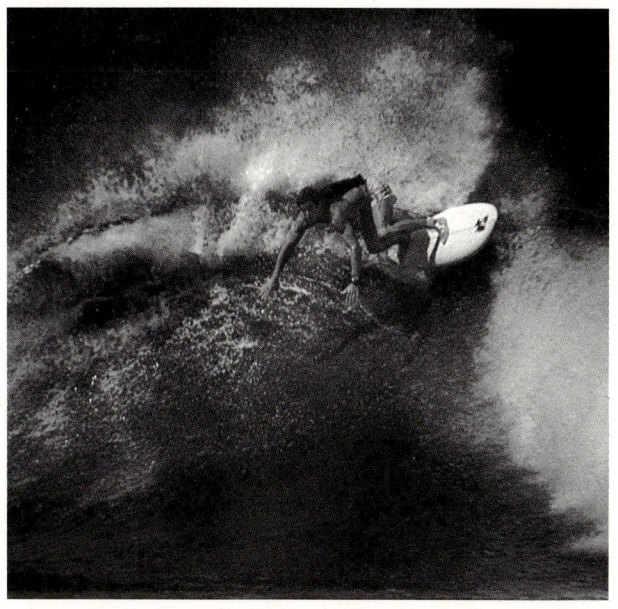

"I've been around the world six times, going to surfing contests. There's not that much money in it — unless you win."

Burton Dean Kerbox

Vital & Not So Vital Statistics
Birthdate: September 25, 1956
Height: 5'9"
Weight: 165 lbs.
Hair: Dirty-blond
Eyes: Blue

Personal Favorites —
Surfing Spots: Jeffrey's Bay, South Africa; Bali
Surfboard: 3 Fin Thrasher (for any wave under eight feet)
Surfing Hero: Jerry Lopez
Color: Blue
Movie: *Raiders of The Lost Ark*
Food: Fresh fish, raw or cooked
Drinks: Heineken beer; fresh-squeezed carrot and orange juice; Kahlúa and coffee
Hangouts: The Fish Market (all the guys that work there are surfers), Bobby McGee's, both in Kailua; The Charthouse, Los Angeles
Ideal Vacation Spot: The Alps, Switzerland, France
Most Beautiful Beach: Bali
TV Shows: Old movies
Car: 320i BMW with tinted windows and a sun roof
Spectator Sport: Tennis — "I love to watch McEnroe, Connors, and Borg."
Hobbies: Photography; windsurfing; skiing
Dress Style: Khaki polo pants with a faded gray sweatshirt — "I like clothes that are 100 percent cotton and comfortable."
Music: Rolling Stones; Men at Work; Eagles; America (Buzzy owns two Sony Walkmans)
Agency: Click, New York City

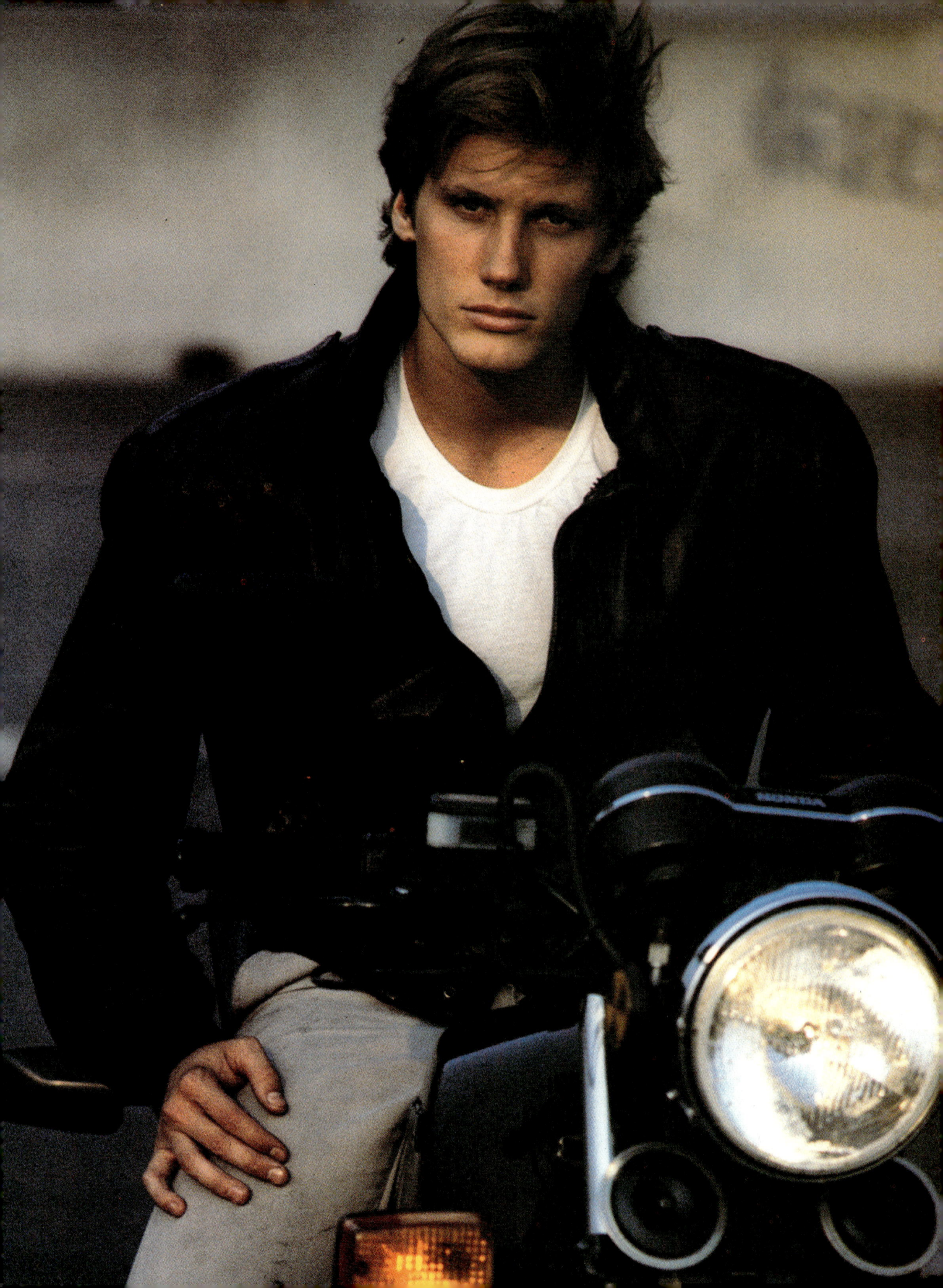

Marcus Abel

"No one can look at my pictures and come to a conclusion about my personality," says Marcus Abel. "I don't see my personality coming through. I look at a picture, and it's not *me*. A photograph is just an image in one hundred twenty-fifth of a second, and it can't capture someone. It can just maybe get something, some quality."

Marcus possesses the blue-eyed, blond-haired American looks that reign in modeling, but he consistently strives to break any stereotypes — about models in general and about himself in particular. "Nobody likes to be categorized," he says. To keep the world off-guard, Marcus may do something rash like cut his long hair short or leave New York and the fashion scene for three months to make a cross-country motorcycle trip. "I'm always changing," he says, "so no photograph is ever going to capture me."

The older of two sons of Estonian immigrants, Marcus is a native New Yorker. He grew up in a Manhattan high-rise that was populated with models who encouraged him to try their profession. "The only reason I started modeling is because I was already in New York," Marcus says. "No way would I have traveled any distance to do it." At the time he started, Marcus was enrolled in film school at New York University, from which he graduated in 1982. To him, modeling was not an exercise in glamor but a way to finance his education and buy some fiscal freedom. Marcus has maintained a nonchalant attitude: "I never could understand how other models busted their asses to do it. Looks are just *there*. I never look as good to myself in real life as I do in my pictures."

Photography is one of Marcus's interests, and, as a model, he has enjoyed firsthand knowledge of the art through exposure to some of the world's most respected photographers. "One of the important things I've learned," he observes, "is what

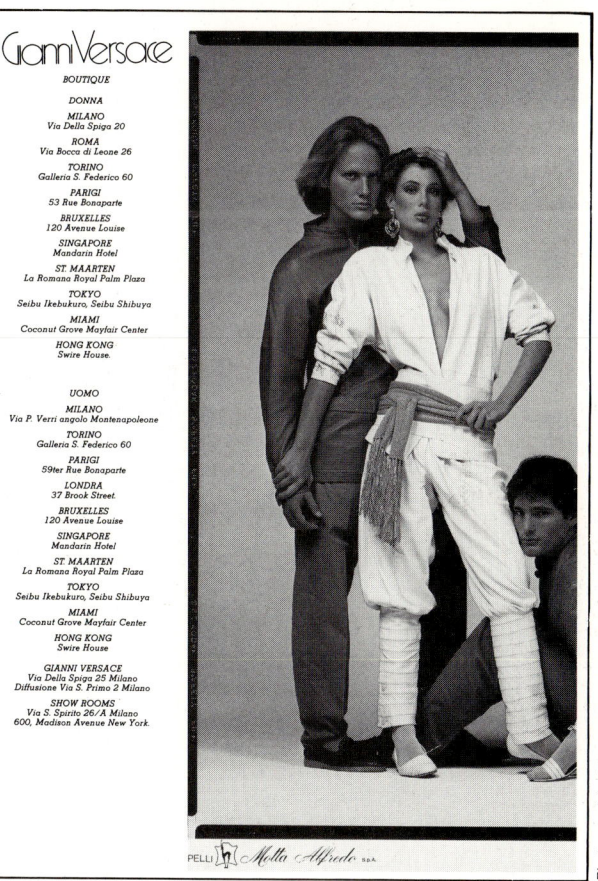

Photograph by Richard Avedon for Gianni Versace

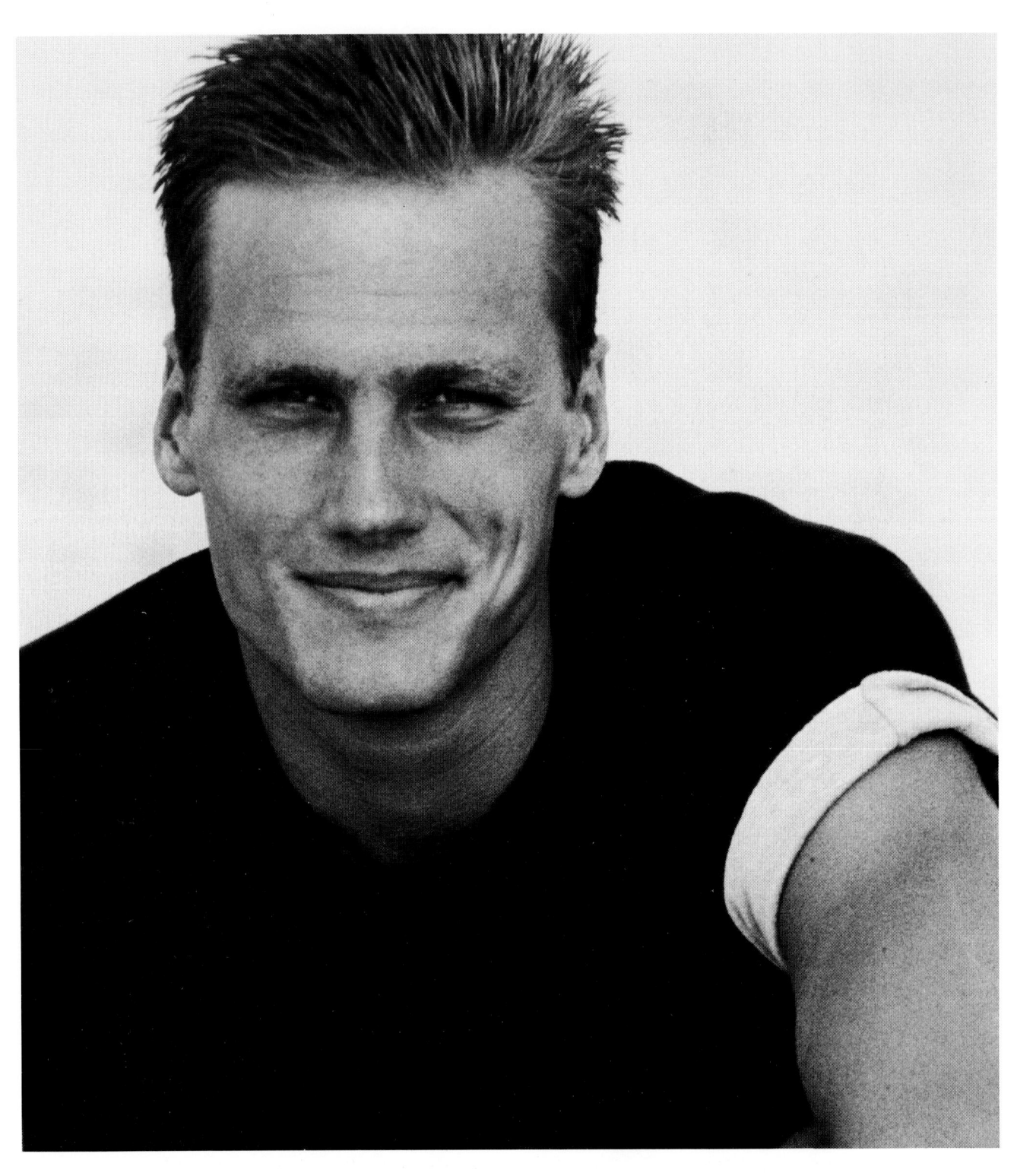

makes a good working environment, which is usually 'do it fast, get it over with quickly.' That's the situation I work best in." The associations with top photographers have been understandably heady and eye-opening. "When I was in school, it was strange, because we'd be talking about a photographer in class, and then I'd be working with him. When you're shooting with Richard Avedon, for instance, you see him in the context of a working person, and not a legend that's studied in schools."

When Marcus isn't racing around town on shoots, he's racing at Bridgehampton and other circuits around the Northeast on his Honda 750 motorcycle, which is probably his most prized possession. "I've always liked motorcycles, but my parents never wanted me to have one. They were trying to protect their offspring or something.

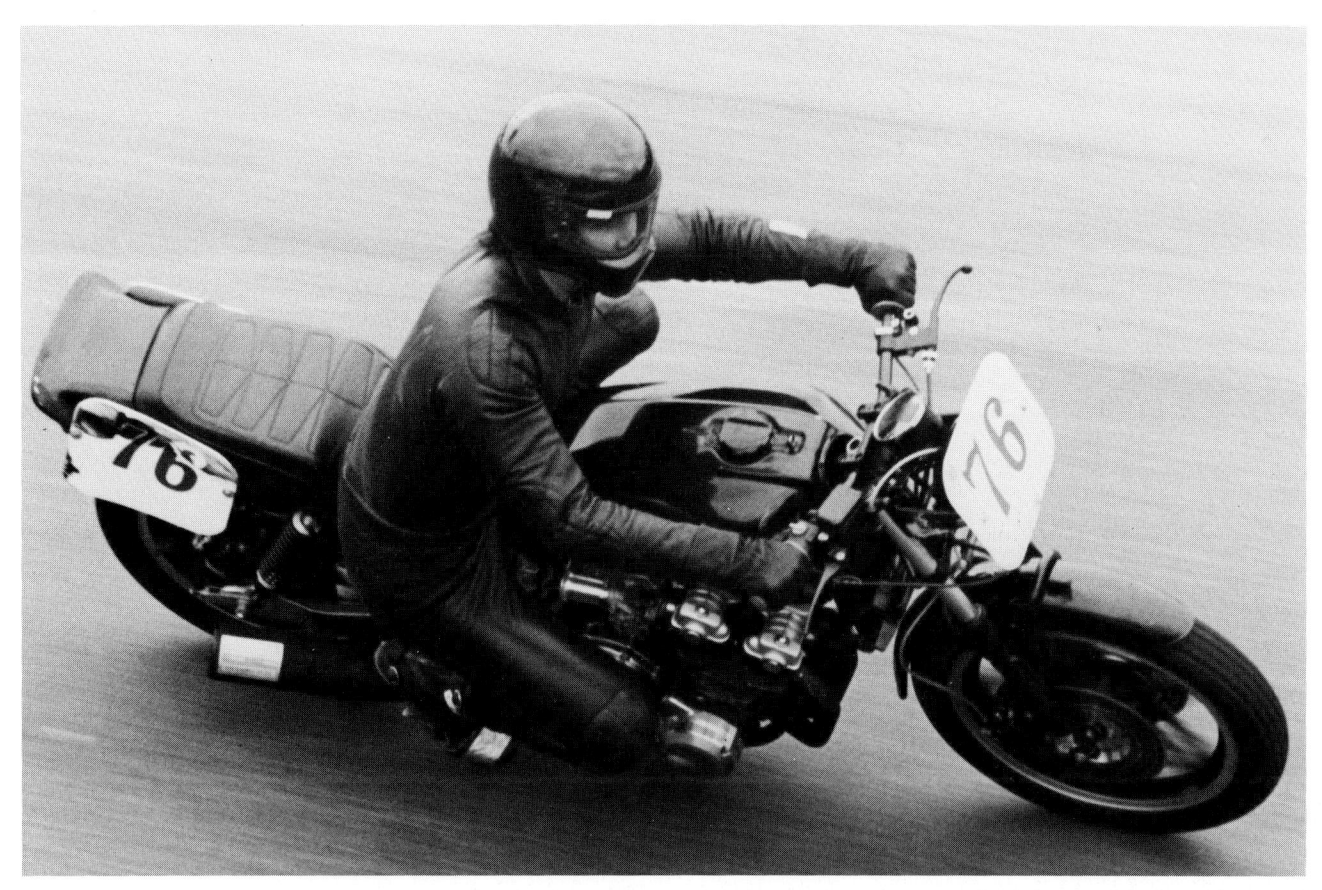

"My energy level is high, but short. I like to do things quickly."

But through modeling, I saved up enough funds to buy one." Marcus has made two cross-country trips on his bike.

Protective of his privacy, Marcus doesn't often partake of the high life that is associated with high fashion. Marcus won't always admit to his profession. "There are emotional things I've had to deal with," he says. "People make one of two assumptions. They are either awed because you're a model or they don't like you because of it. It bothers me that someone might instantly dislike me because of modeling." Marcus currently lives on Manhattan's West Side in an unpretentious apartment well suited to his modesty. Scattered around the apartment are copies of motorcycle and camera arts magazines.

Marcus is still contemplating what profession to enter after modeling, with photography the front-runner. But he is confident of success in whatever he picks. "I've never doubted that whatever I did, I would be successful. I think it's my upbringing. My parents came off the boat, and now they're well-to-do." Marcus doesn't want to limit himself, however, to a single career, a single choice, a single outlook. "I like things to change," he says. "I get bored quickly. If things become the same old routine, it's not intriguing."

Marcus Abel
Vital & Not So Vital Statistics
Birthdate: August 3, 1959
Height: 6'
Weight: 180 lbs.
Hair: Blond
Eyes: Blue-gray
Personal Favorites —
Time of Day: Early morning
Motorcycle: Suzuki GS1100
Car: Ferrari 275 GTB4
Drinks: Cranberry juice; milk
Color: Black
Movie: *Badlands,* directed by Terrence Malick
Actor: Marlon Brando
TV Shows: *Ugly George;* Cable News Network; ESPN Sports
Photographers: Joel Mayerweitz; Les Krims
Vacation Spot: Saint Martin, West Indies
Hobbies: Motorcycle racing; volleyball; photography
Hangouts: Bridgehampton racetrack
Town: New York City
Restaurants: Hunan Cafe, Kamon, both in New York City
Type of Woman: "Ultimately her personality, but I like nice lips."
Socks: Argyle
Designers: Gianni Versace; Calvin Klein
Agency: Zoli, New York City

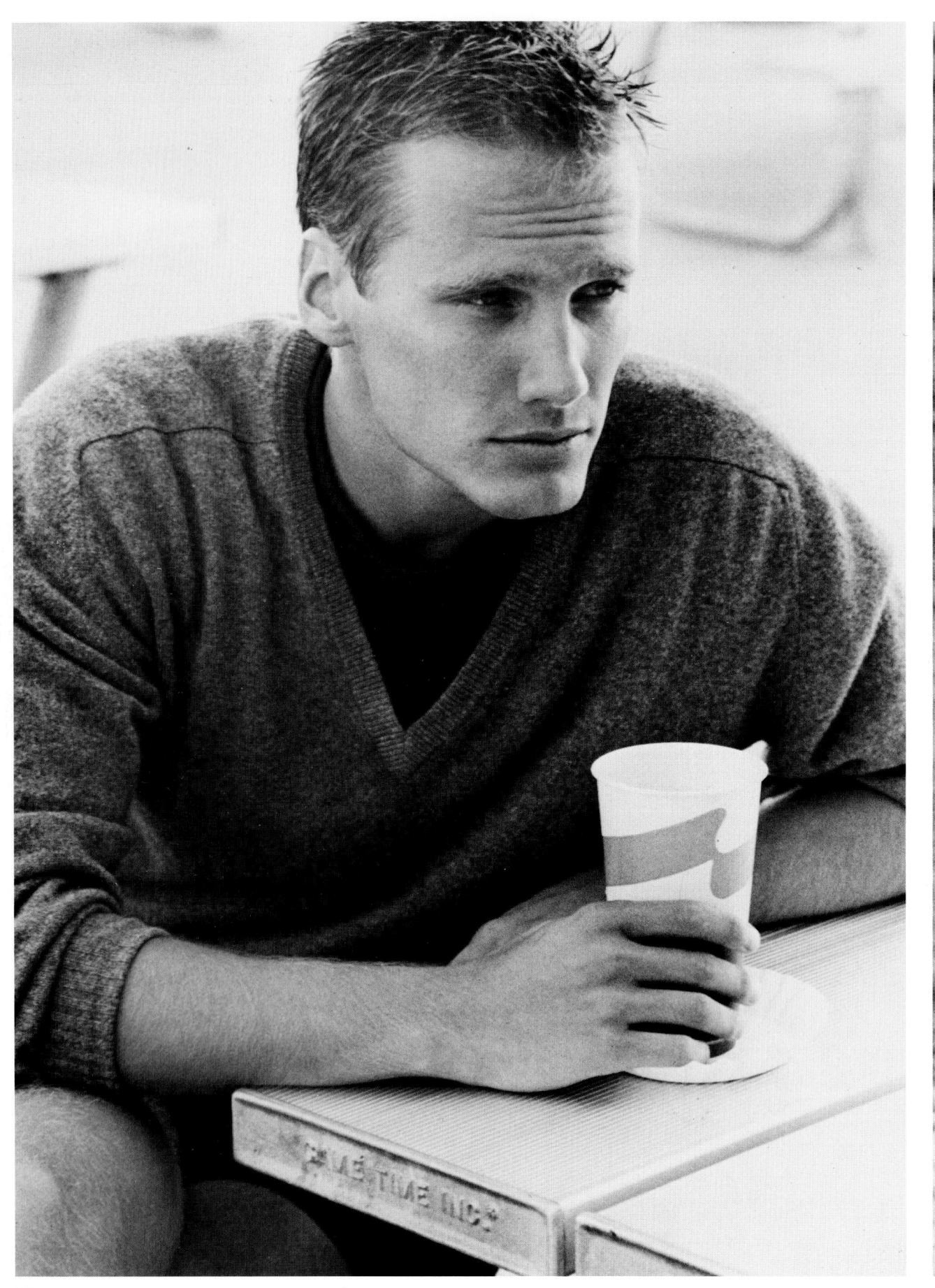

63

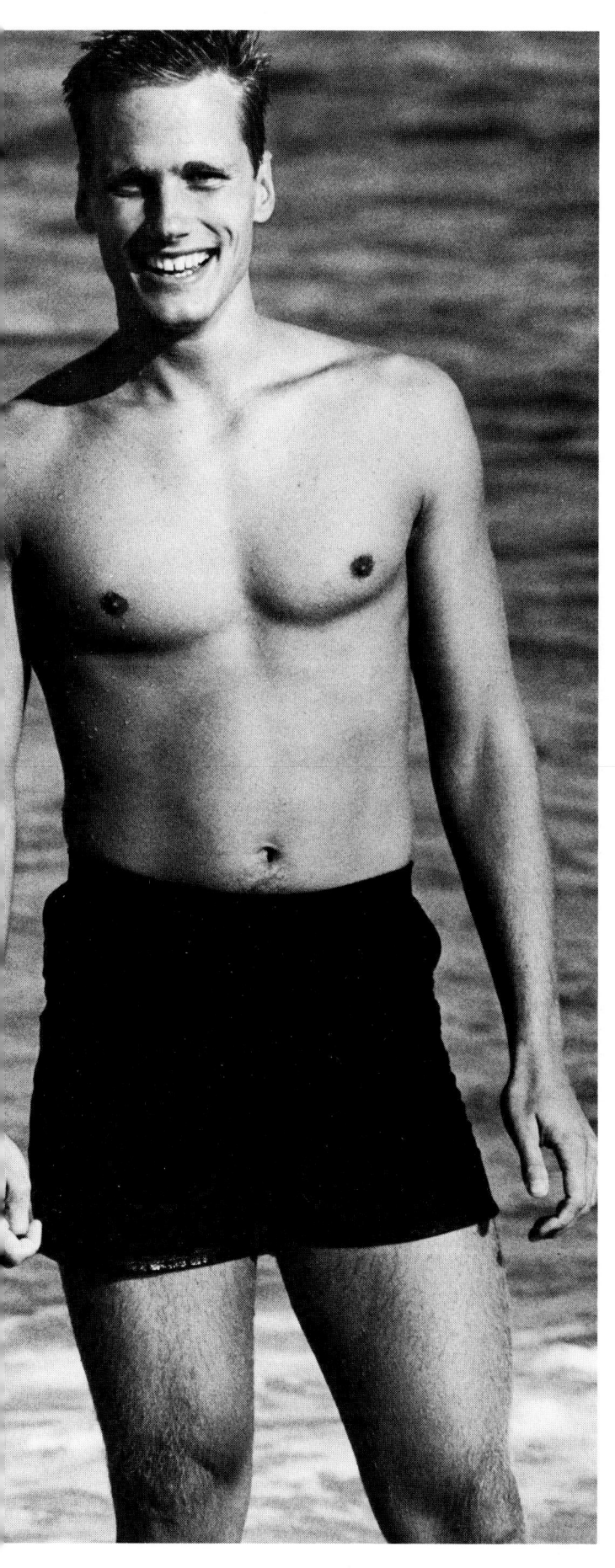

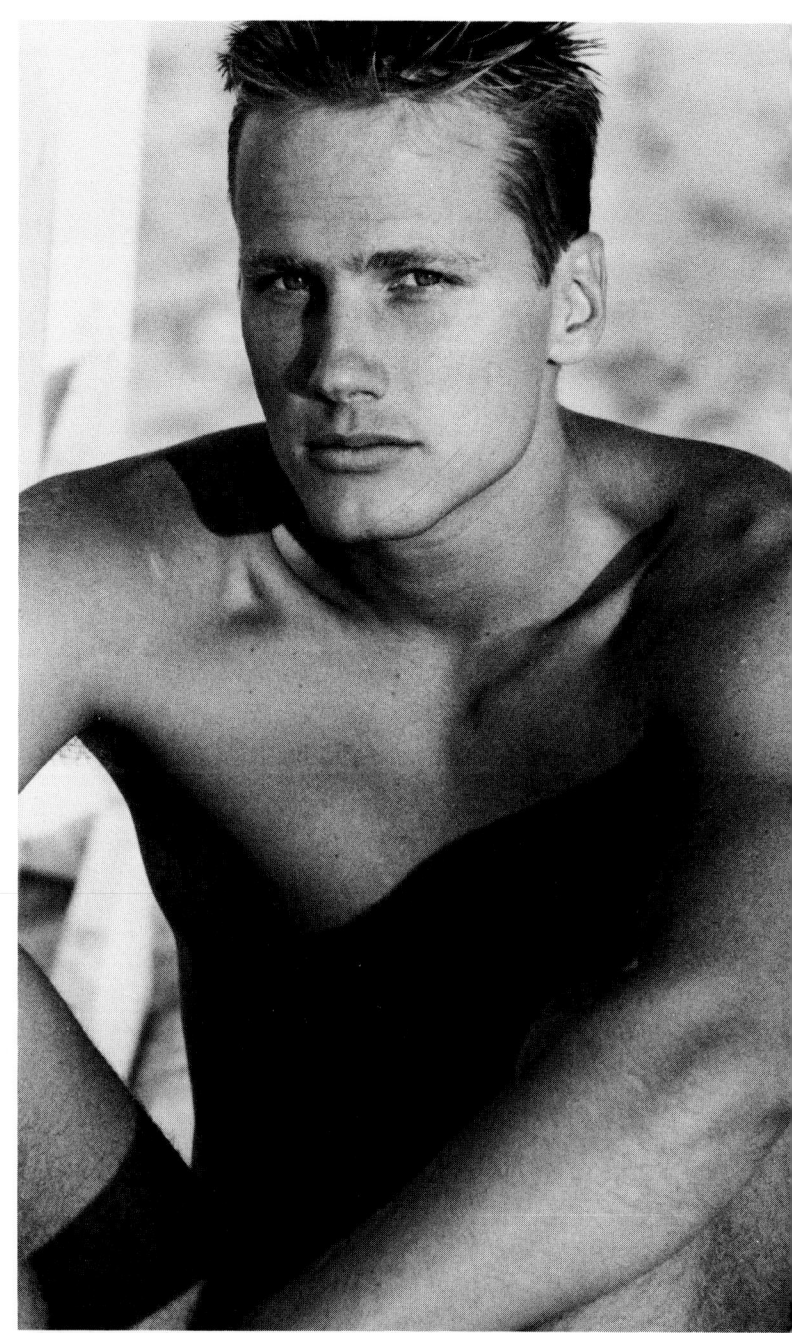

Andrew Smith

The ultimate California beach boys, Andrew Smith and St. John Smith have caused many a double take. The Smiths aren't the only brother act in modeling, but they are the most in demand. The youngest sons in a close-knit California family of four boys and two girls, the Smiths have appeared in several ads together, including a popular one for Coppertone. Though their similar looks may put the pair in competition with one another, each enjoys having a brother in the business. "It's great. It really works to our advantage," says St. John, called Sinjin, who is a year older than Andrew. "If we're up for the same job, often a client will use us both. Or if Andrew is in New York and I'm in California, we'll reap the benefits from each other's jobs. Somebody in California may ask for Andrew but use me if he's not around."

If the blond-haired, blue-eyed, muscle-toned brothers conjure up images of sand, surf, and endless summers, it's no accident. For these guys, the beach is their home away from home. Born and raised in the sun-and-surf capital, Santa Monica, California, the Smiths grew up beside the ocean, and they still spend as much time there as possible. "I can't stand to be inside if the sun is shining," explains Sinjin. "I've *got* to get out and play volleyball and exercise."

Appropriately enough, the Smiths were discovered right on the beach where they perfected their surfing, sunning, and swimming skills. In late October 1980, Andrew was running on the beach when he passed a fashion shoot under way near the edge of the water. The photographer, Herb Rits, asked Andrew if he would be interested in working for *GQ*. Rits took some Polaroid shots of Andrew and then showed the pictures to fellow photographer Bruce Weber, who was in town looking for new faces for *GQ*. "That night," recalls Andrew, "Donald Sterzin, the art director for *GQ*, called me up and asked to see me the next day. I met with him and Bruce Weber. I asked a lot of questions; I wanted to make sure the pictures would be a fair representation of me." As Sinjin recalls, "Bruce Weber asked Andrew if he had any other friends with similar looks. Andrew mentioned my name along with a few others. That's how I got in." The brothers debuted in the February 1981 issue of *GQ*. "That was basically our ticket into the business," says Sinjin. They were immediately besieged with offers; Andrew was offered a trip to New York, Sinjin a trip to Haiti.

Andrew, who graduated from UCLA with a degree in psychology, is an adventurous, fun-loving guy who likes to snow ski in the winter and windsurf and play beach volleyball the rest of the year. "I like people who are now happy and jovial, then quiet and shy," says Andrew. "People that have fun and are active." And he conveys that quality in his much-admired photos. "I try and project my self-image," he says. "Most of my shots deal with smiling and happiness, which is good, because I like to laugh and have fun."

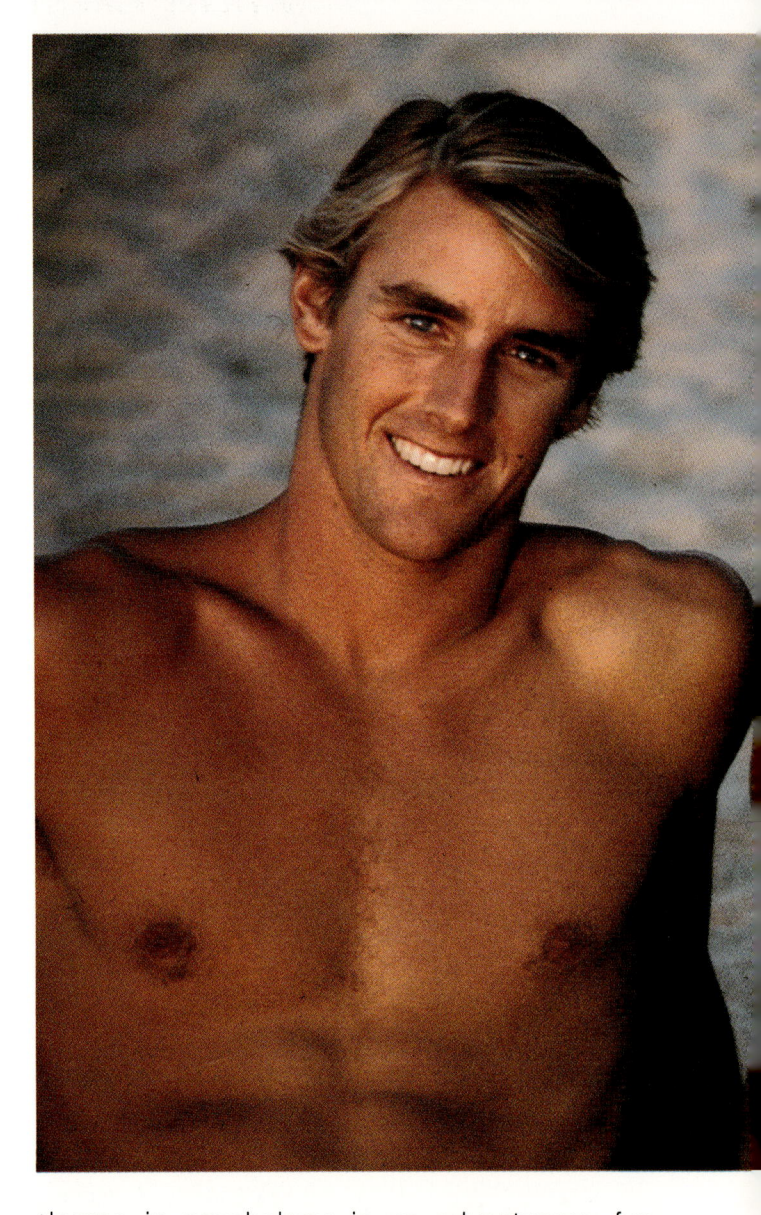

Andrew's all-American looks and carefree smile are often mistaken for Michael Ives's. And Ives has experienced the same problem. Once, when Michael was sitting at an outdoor cafe, two young women approached and asked him, "Excuse me,

Sinjin Smith

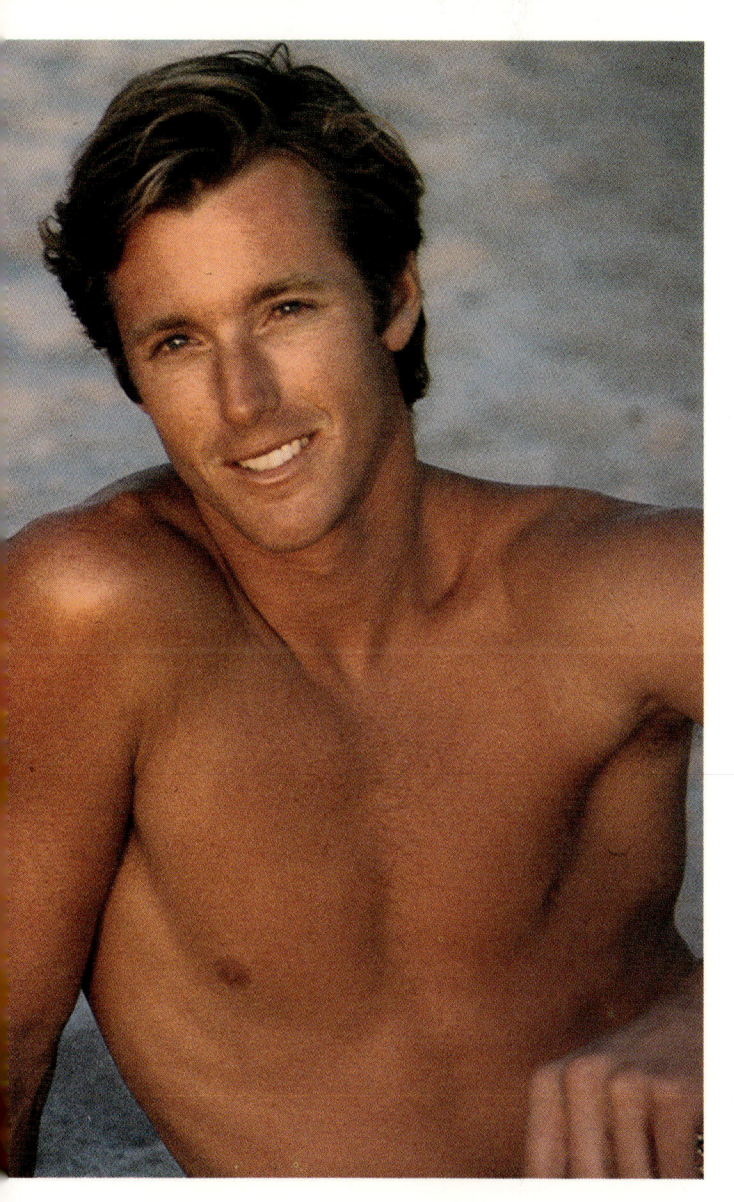

Chaps by Ralph Lauren:
Drawing a Fine Line When it Comes to Stripes

The Parallel Perspective in a rich choice of eight summer colors

Capturing the elusive qualities of summer in Ralph's polo shirt for Chaps. At home on South Hampton's Jobs Lane. Equally at ease at Yankee Stadium. Here, from the collection of candy stripes in raspberry, kelly, turquoise, pink, navy, red, citron or electric blue. All with contrasting collars and ribbed cuffs. Sizes S,M,L,XL. 24.00

Chaps by Ralph Lauren on 1, New York. And in all our fashion stores, Jenkintown included.

Chaps by Ralph Lauren at bloomingdale's men's store

are you Andrew Smith?" Michael answered, "No, but I'm a model too." Disbelieving and disappointed, the girls looked him up and down and said sarcastically, "Sure."

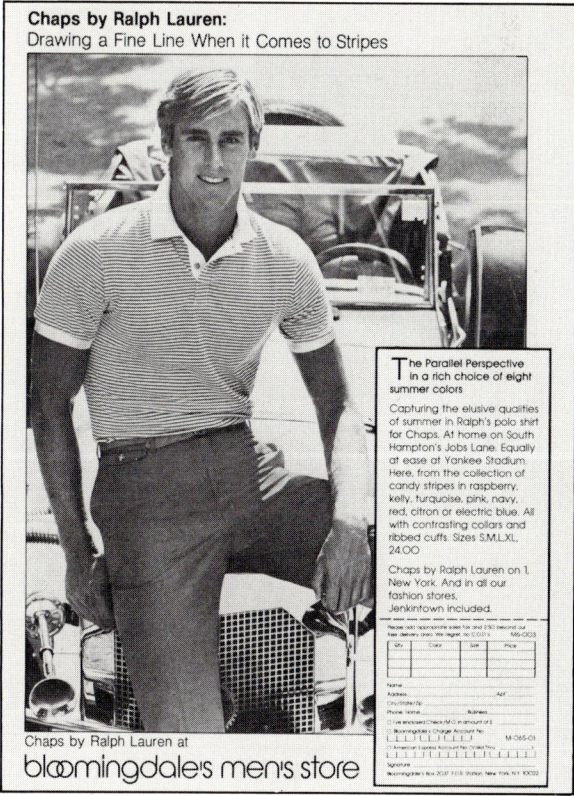

Sinjin majored in economics at UCLA, where he received a scholarship for his sensational volleyball skills. An expert player, Sinjin began honing his talent on the court in his backyard as a child. He started to play competitively in high school, a Jesuit institution that all the Smith brothers attended. Sinjin's room is covered with trophies won over the years During his senior year at UCLA, Sinjin was recruited for the U.S. national volleyball team, and he has traveled to China, Brazil, Japan, and Bulgaria to participate in international tournaments. (Andrew, who was also a top player, gave up competitive volleyball to concentrate on modeling.) "My first priority right now," says Sinjin, "is to play on the U.S. volleyball team in the 1984 Olympics. That's why I'm in Los Angeles." Eyeing the long-sought gold medal, Sinjin does some sort of exercise every day. "Staying in shape is very important for me," he says. "On the national volleyball team, you work out six hours a day. When I'm in New York and can't exercise on the beach, I go crazy. I've had to settle for jumping rope in a trash room while it was snowing outside because it was the only place where the ceilings were high enough." At volleyball tournaments on California beaches, T-shirts with Sinjin's image silk-screened on the back are sold to eager fans. Sinjin is more reserved and perhaps a touch more conservative than his younger brother, but that doesn't diminish his sexiness. Sinjin is a disciplined type, who sets his sights on a goal and then focuses all his energy on achieving it. "Everything I've gotten or done well at, I've spent a lot of time on," says Sinjin. "It might seem like it's come really easy, but in reality, it's taken a lot of work."

When it comes to fashion, the Smiths prefer casual beach clothes and corduroy pants to jeans. "My general rule about clothes," says Sinjin, "is if it's in style, I don't wear it." Andrew agrees: "I *have* to dress comfortably. I seldom wear the clothes that I model. And despite what everyone thinks, they don't give us the clothes we model." To stay in shape for modeling, Andrew plays tennis as well as volleyball. "I can't work out with weights," he says, "because I get too bulky and then I never fit the clothes."

When in town, both men live with their mother and youngest sister at home in Brentwood, California. The Brentwood house has a very popular Jacuzzi, and Andrew and Sinjin are looking at other property to build on. For the future, Andrew plans to continue modeling "as long as I can," and then explore a job in money management. After the Olympics, Sinjin would like to get into acting, if opportunity beckons. "But male models can work for a long time," he observes, "and I plan to take advantage of it while I can." Whatever careers they next pursue, Andrew and Sinjin want to make sure they have plenty of free time for the beach. Nine-to-five routines are washouts. Says Andrew, "I don't ever want to spend all my time behind a desk." Spoken like a true beach boy.

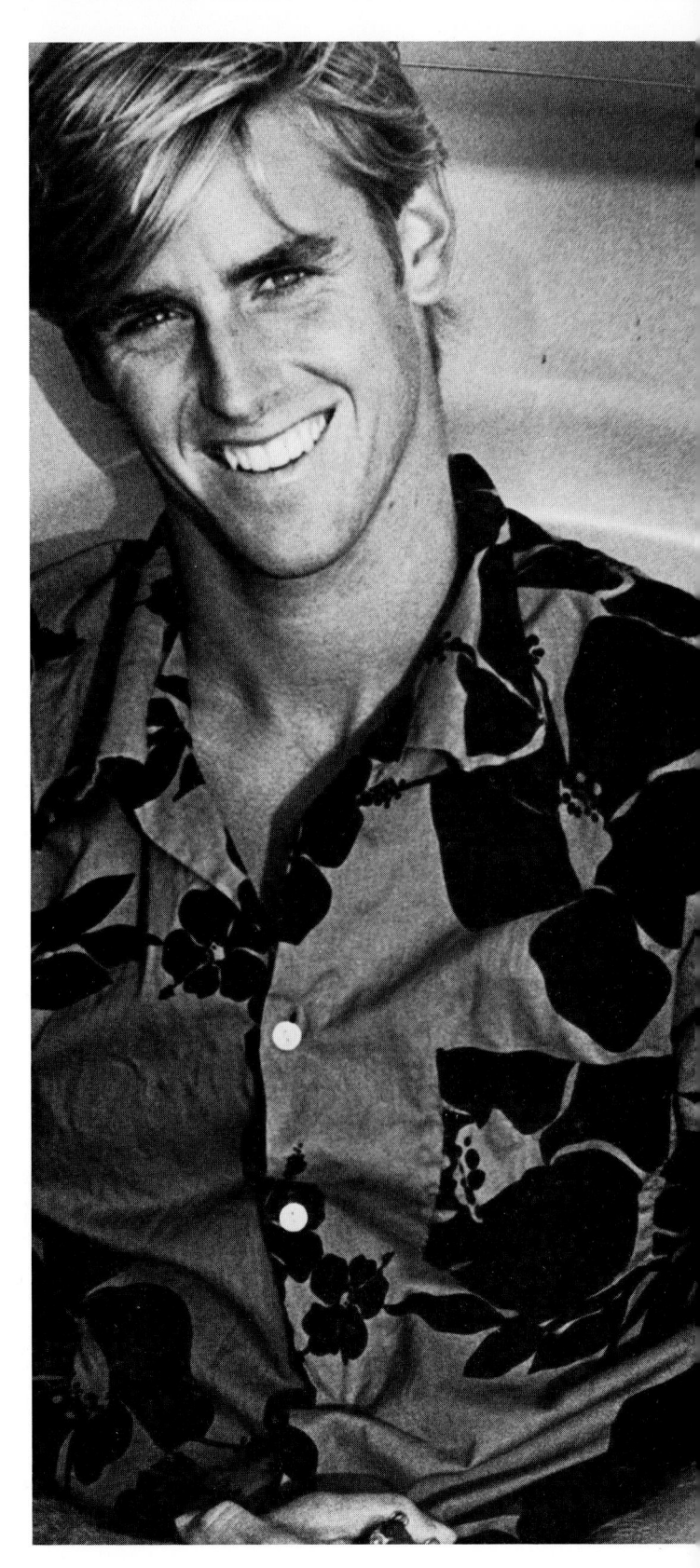

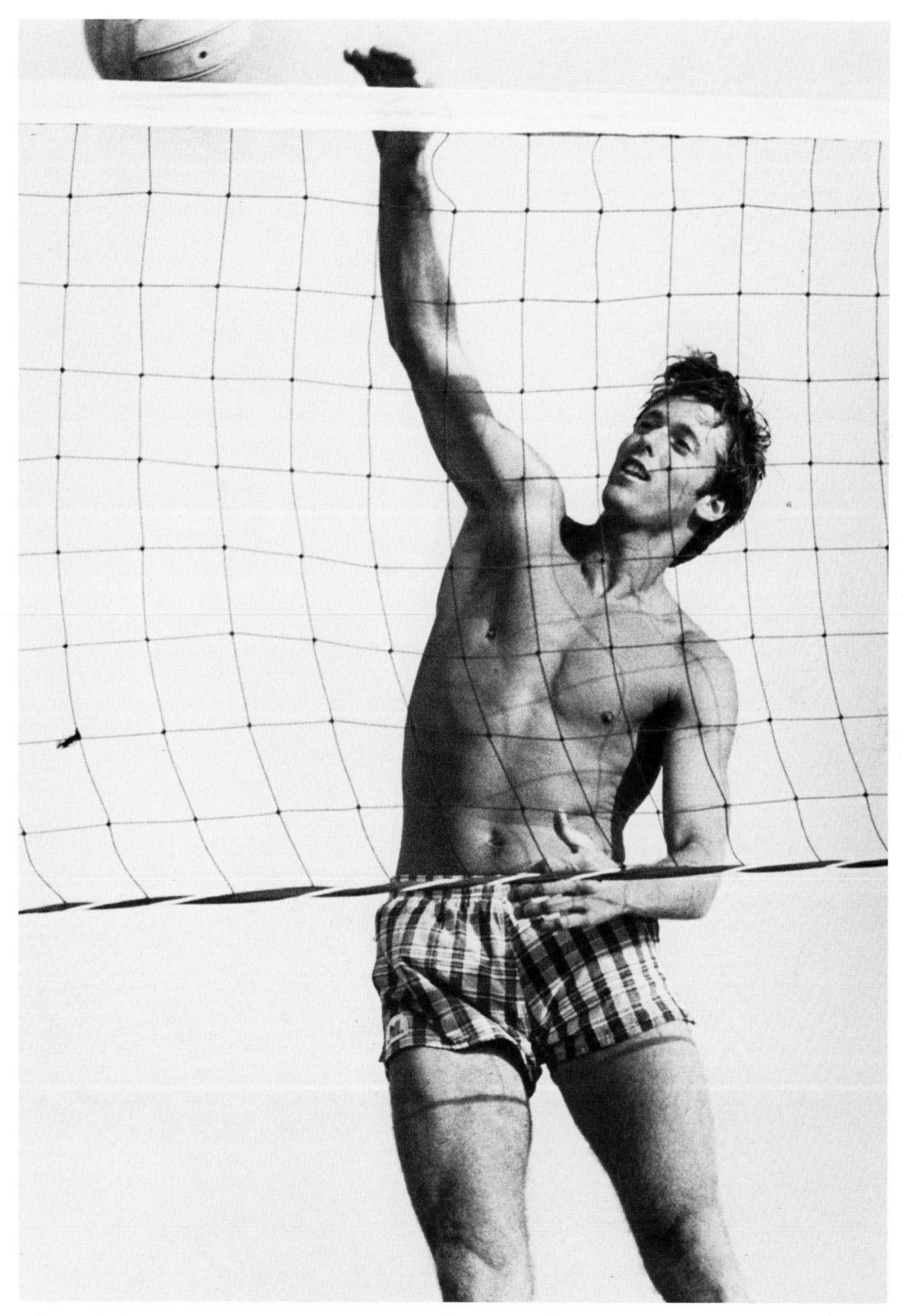

"It may look easy — but everything I've achieved, I've worked hard for."

68

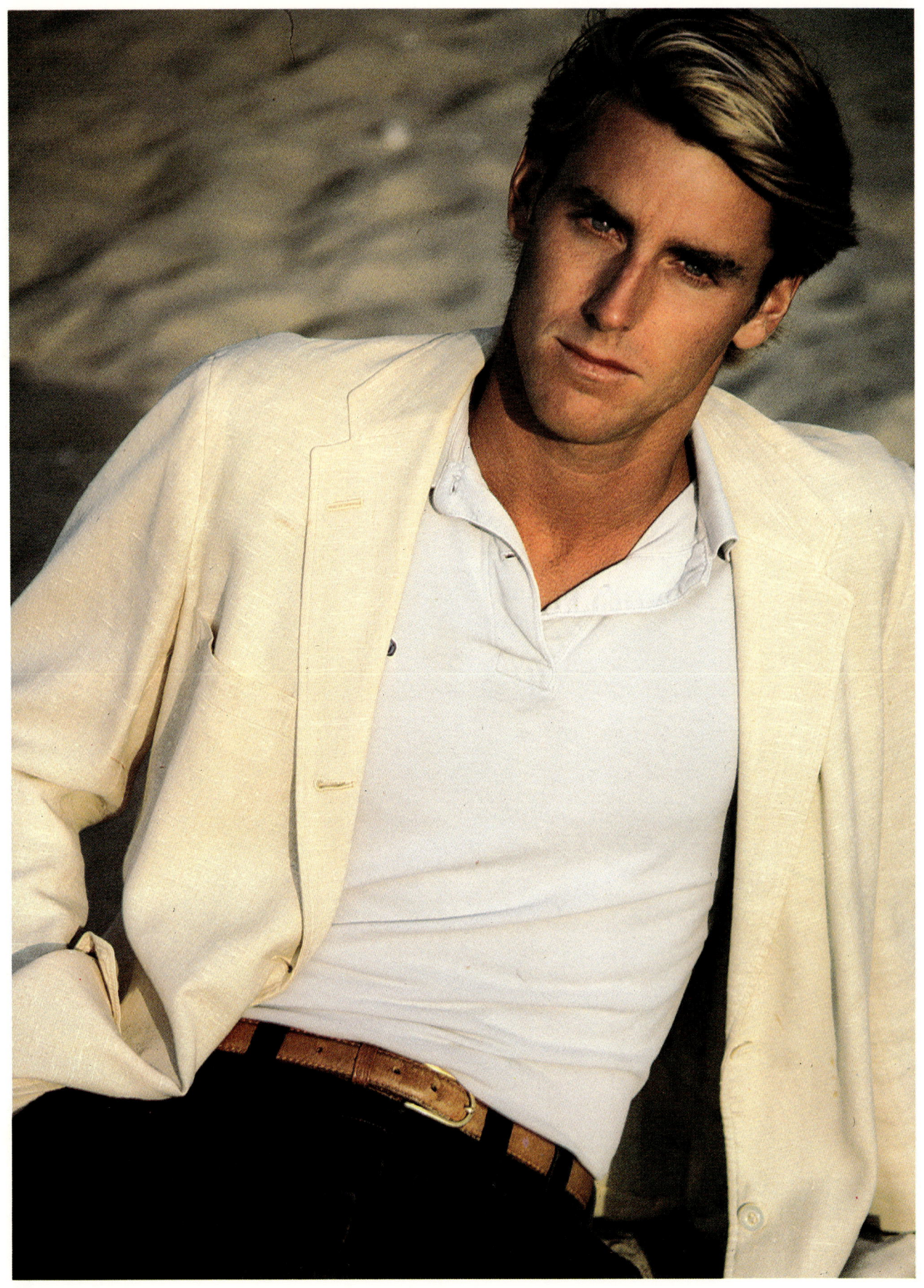

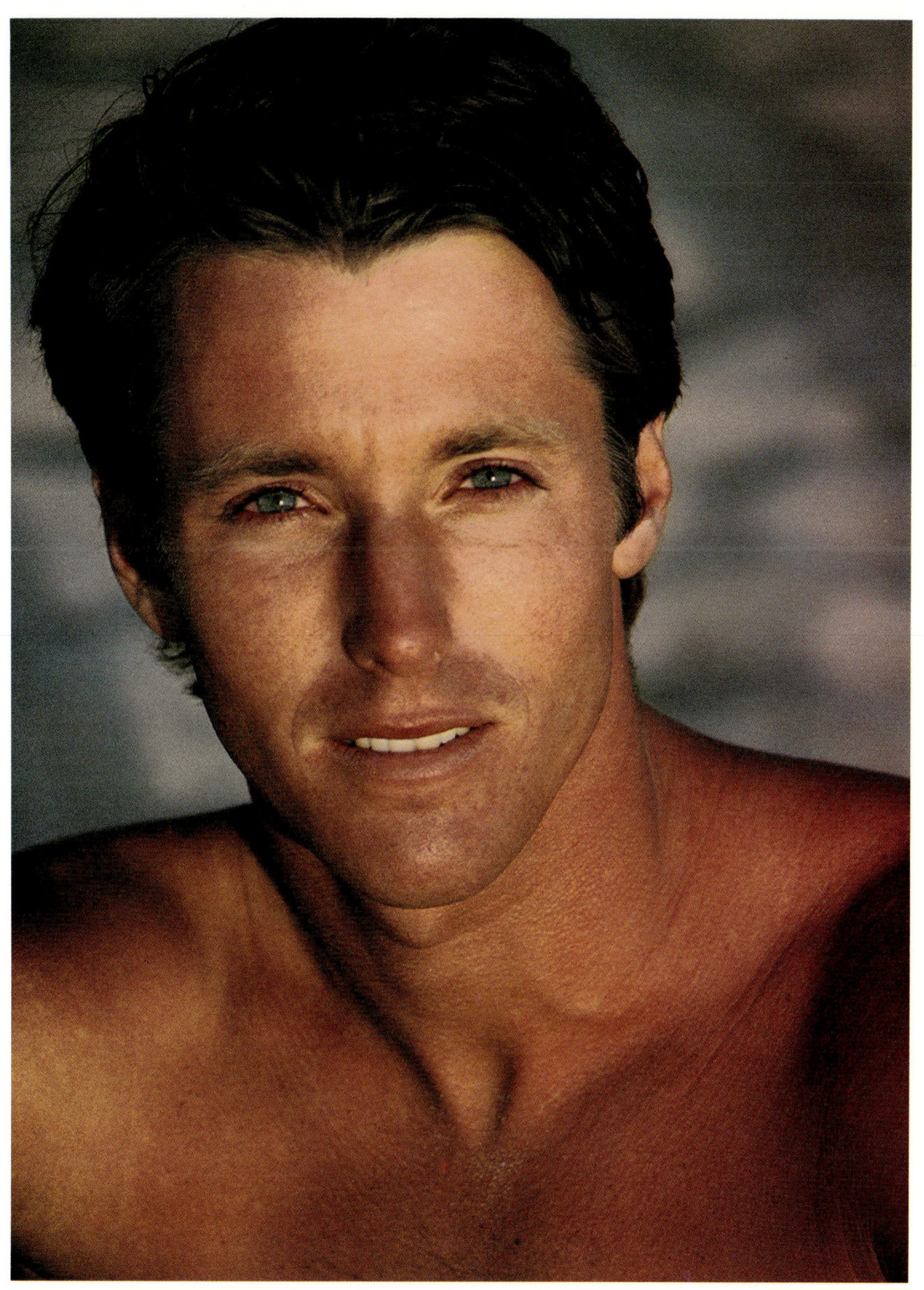

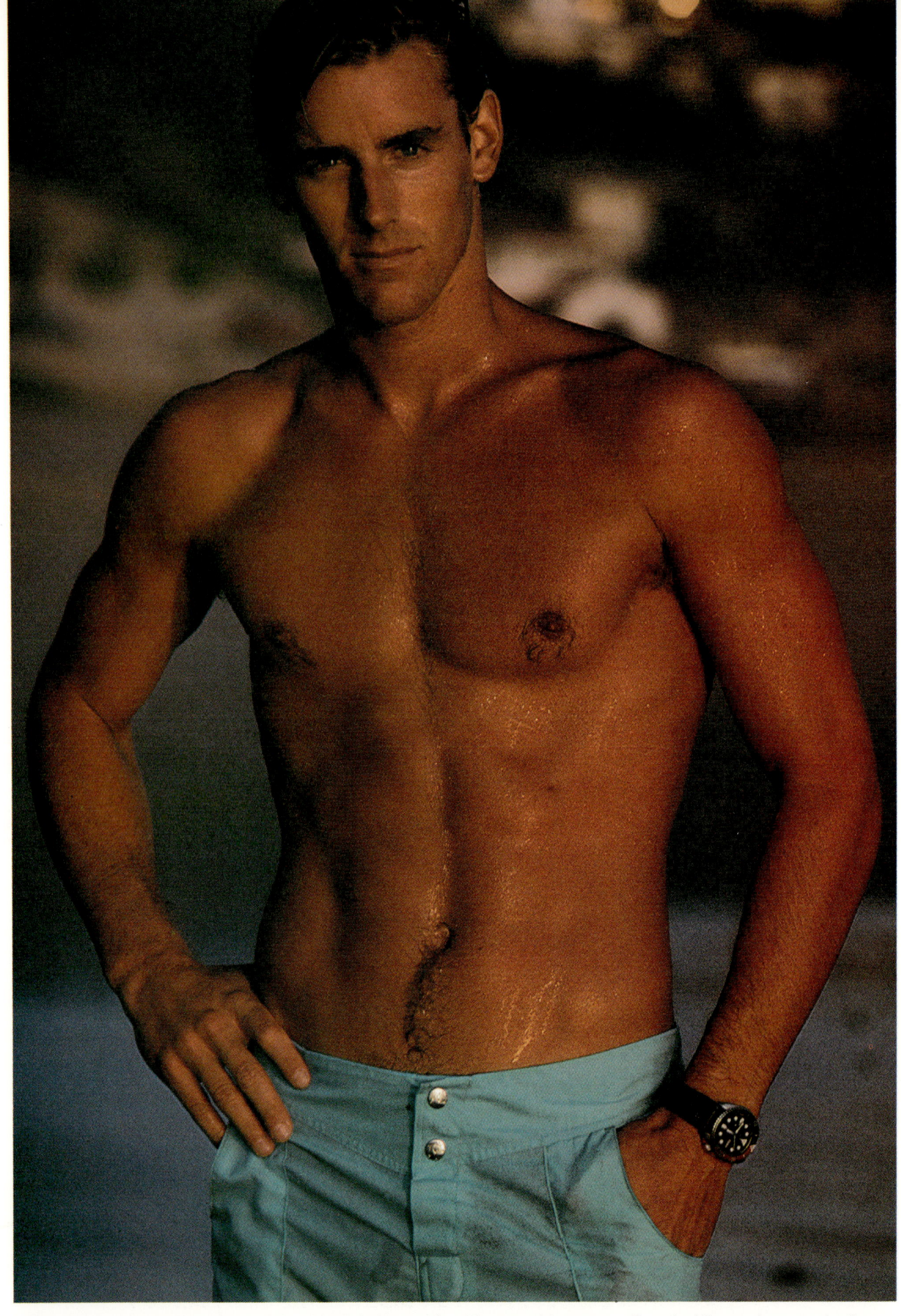

"The most important thing about relationships is being comfortable around the person. If you feel like you know each other, it makes things so much easier."

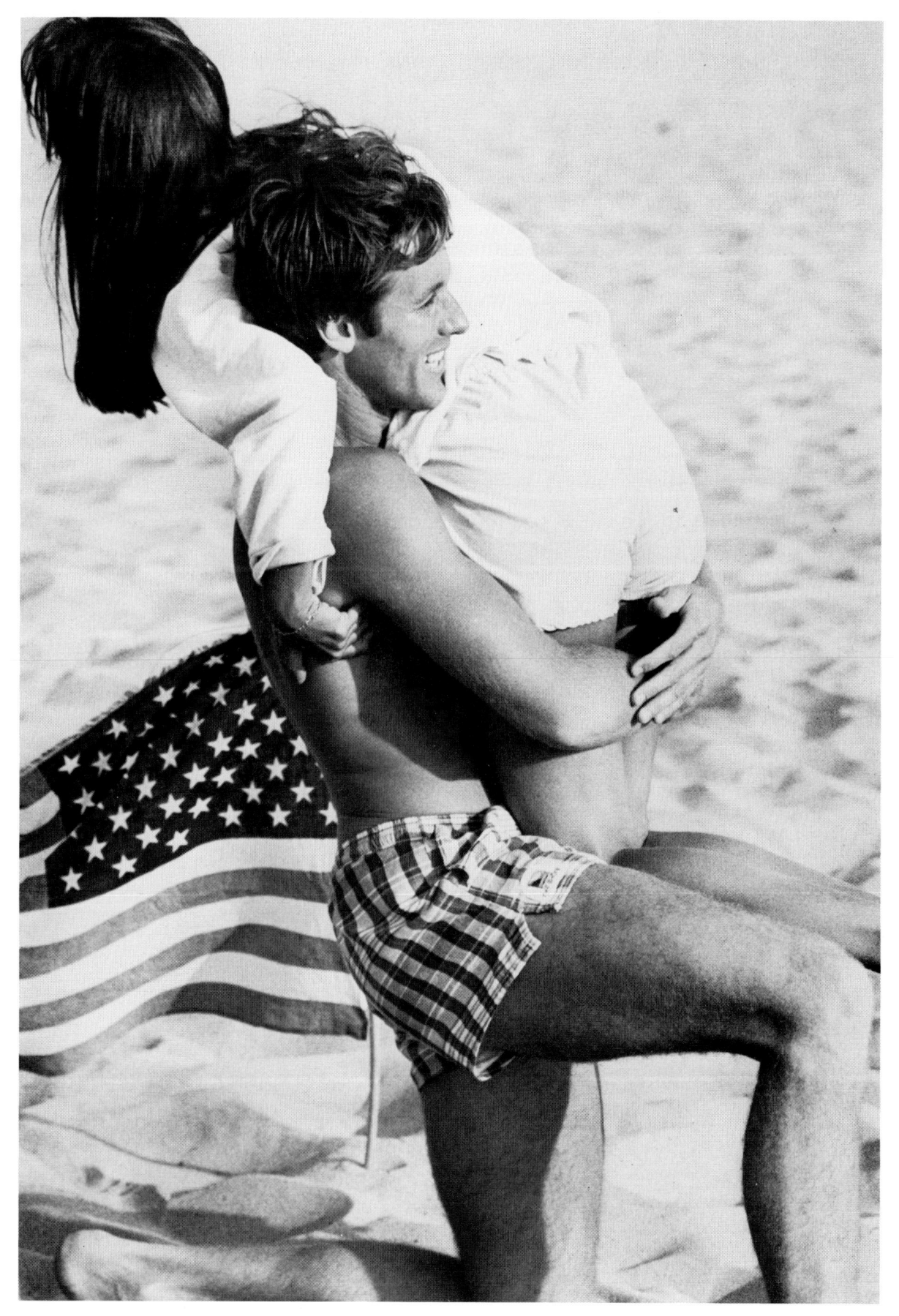

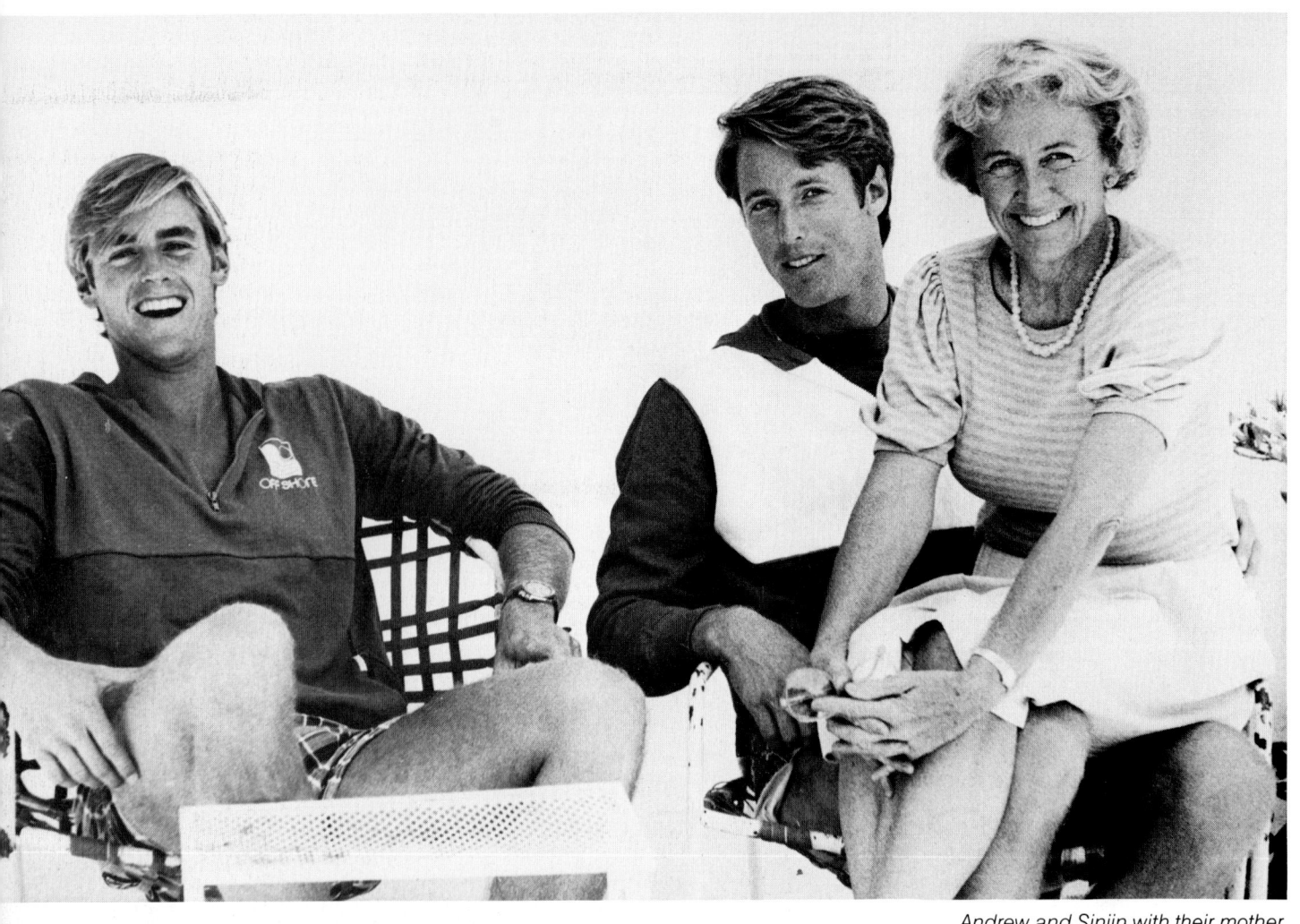

Andrew and Sinjin with their mother.

> My whole itinerary is health and exercise. My favorite things for staying in shape are volleyball, surfing, windsurfing, and playing tennis. — Andrew

Andrew Smith
Vital & Not So Vital Statistics
Birthdate: May 22, 1958
Height: 6'2"
Weight: 185 lbs.
Hair: Blond
Eyes: Blue

Personal Favorites —
Time of Day: Evenings, when the sun sets
Town: New York City
Movie: *Raiders of the Lost Ark*
Actor: Clark Gable
Actress: Mae West
TV Show: *M*A*S*H*
Vacation Spots: Virgin Islands; Aspen, Colorado
Drink: Cranberry-apple juice
Music: Rolling Stones; Flock of Seagulls
Hobbies: Volleyball; windsurfing; snow skiing
Designers: Ralph Lauren; Alan Flusser
Most Memorable Moment: "Being discovered on the beach and being put on the cover of *GQ*"
Ambition: "To become the next James Bond in the movies"
Agencies: Nina Blanchard, Los Angeles
Click, New York City

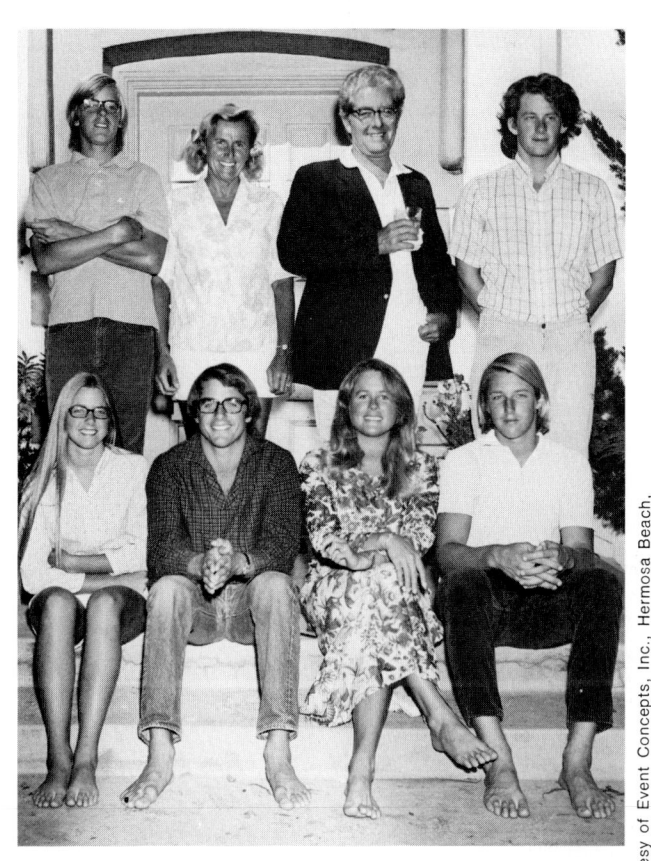

The Smith Family: (top, l. to r.) Andrew, Mary-Lou (mother), James Celestine (father), Paul; (bottom, l. to r.) Rosebud, Beaver, Georgie, Sinjin.

St. John Smith
Vital & Not So Vital Statistics
Birthdate: May 7, 1957
Height: 6'1"
Weight: 185 lbs.
Hair: Dark blond
Eyes: Blue
Personal Favorites —
Town: Santa Monica
Cartoon: *Road Runner*
Actors: Errol Flynn; Burt Lancaster; Clint Eastwood
Actress: Shirley Temple
Movie: *Raiders of the Lost Ark*
Snack: Wheatberry toast with jack cheese, tomatoes, lettuce, and mayonnaise
Drink: Coconut-pineapple drink
Music: Rolling Stones; Robert Palmer
Color: Blue
Designer: Calvin Klein; North Shore beachwear
Hobbies: Beach volleyball; tennis; surfing; racquetball; golf
Ambition: "To win a gold with the national volleyball team"
Agencies: Nina Blanchard, Los Angeles
Click, New York City

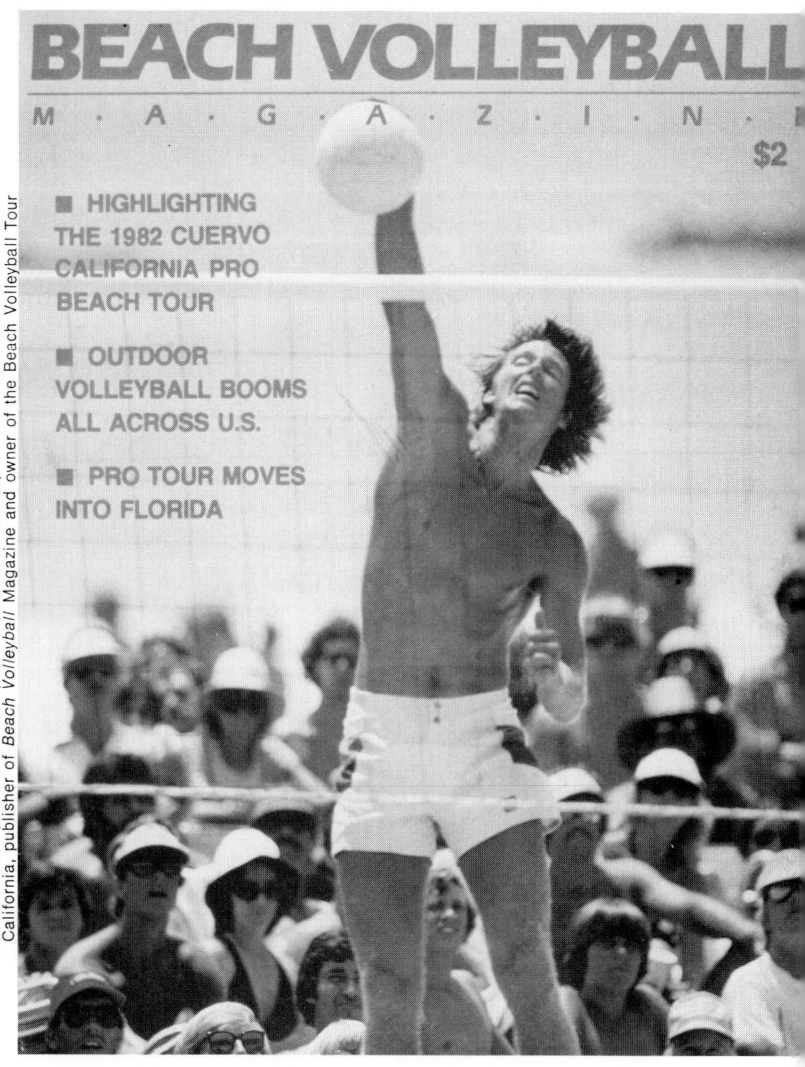

Photo courtesy of Event Concepts, Inc., Hermosa Beach, California, publisher of *Beach Volleyball* Magazine and owner of the Beach Volleyball Tour

BEACH VOLLEYBALL
M·A·G·A·Z·I·N·E
$2

- HIGHLIGHTING THE 1982 CUERVO CALIFORNIA PRO BEACH TOUR
- OUTDOOR VOLLEYBALL BOOMS ALL ACROSS U.S.
- PRO TOUR MOVES INTO FLORIDA

"Until the Olympics are over, I take every day as it comes. I just take advantage of what's available to me. Modeling has been very good to me."

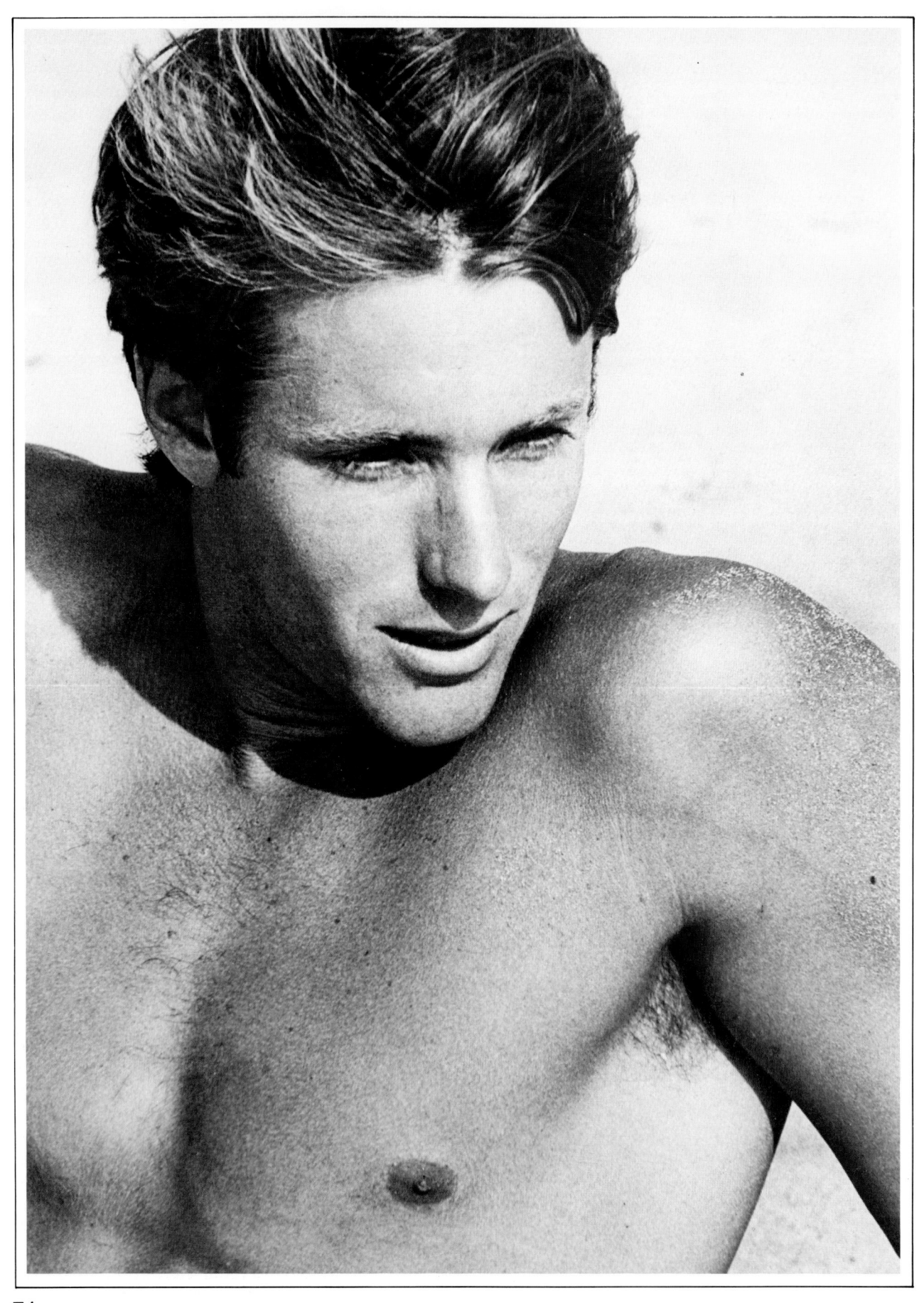

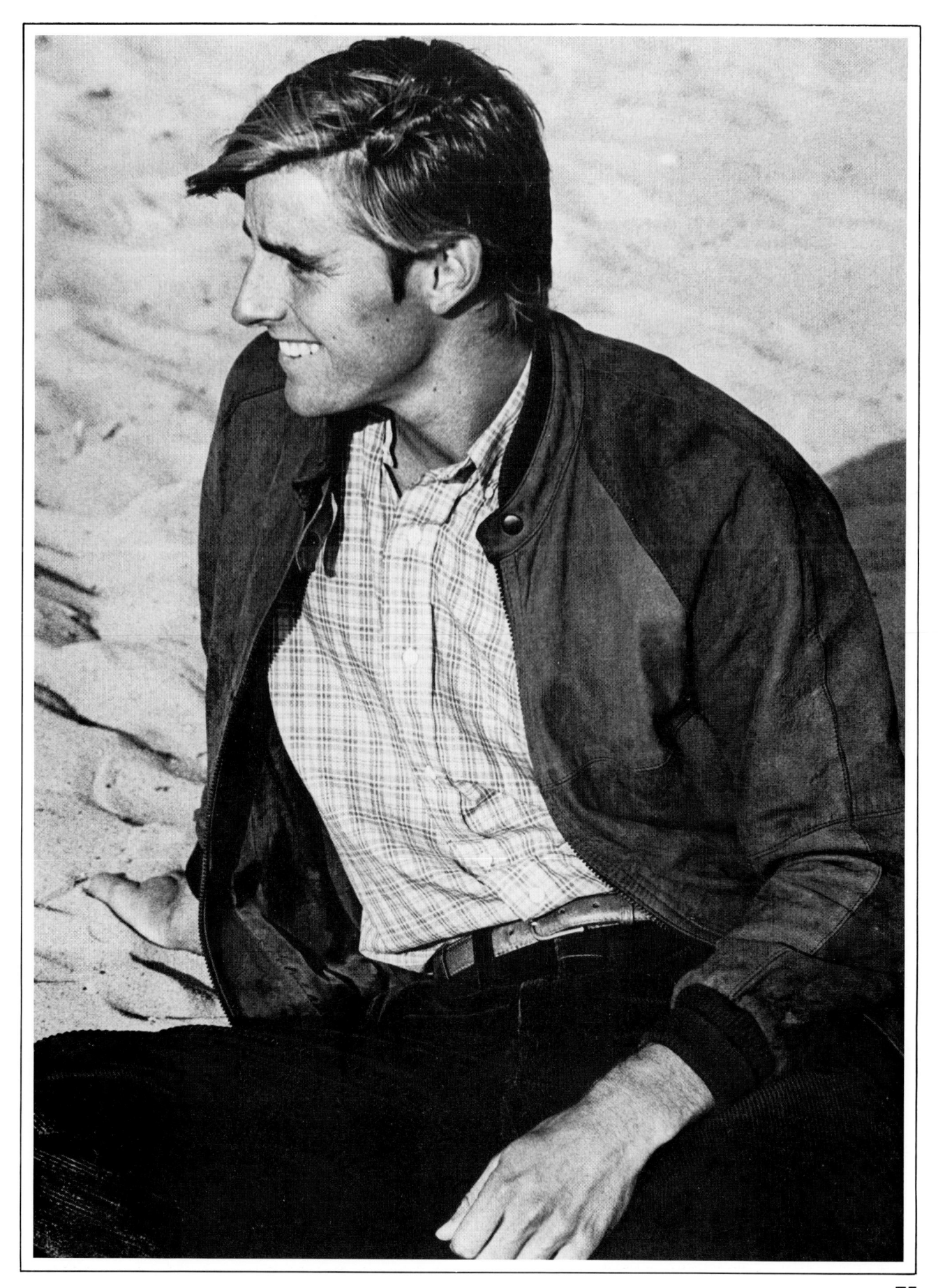

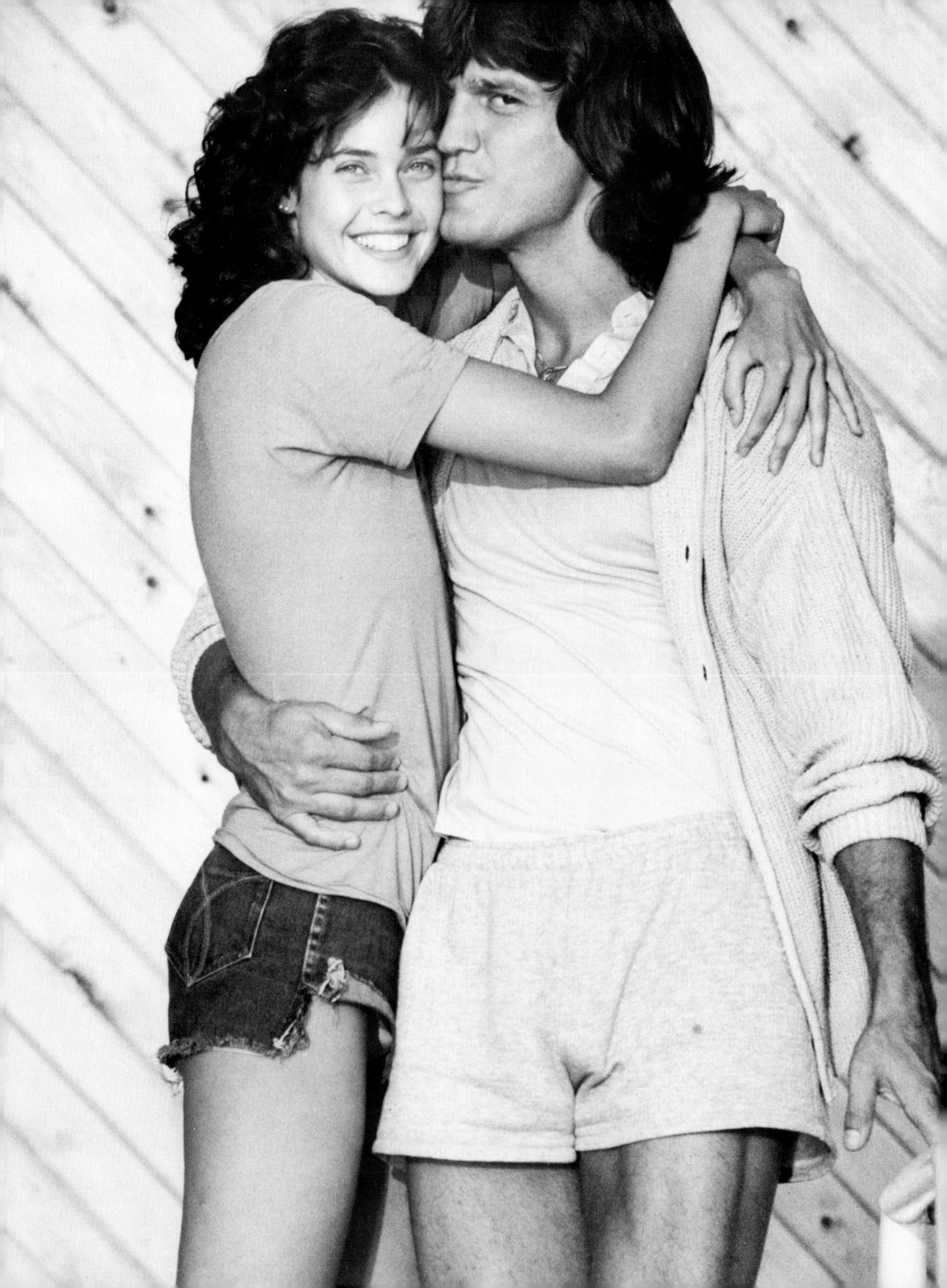

Ron Greschner

To fans of the New York Rangers hockey team, Ron Greschner is a streak of defensive fury, a veritable speed demon. To fans of the New York Rangers' popular commercial for Sasson jeans, Greschner is a streak of intense sexuality. But off the ice and away from the camera, Gresch, as he is known, is a hulking Prince Valiant from up north, a shy, good-hearted Canadian character who's got a flash in his eyes to match his flash on the ice. Full-time athlete, part-time model, good-time guy. Gresch is his own hat trick.

Ron has, quite literally, spent a lifetime in pursuit of the puck. His father is a Czechoslovakian immigrant, his mother a Canadian native, and Ron was born in the small town of Goodsoil, Saskatchewan, Canada. "The only thing further north is the North Pole," he says. Gresch's father bought him a pair of skates at age three. "In that town, you just opened your back door to skate. There were only two things to do in town, play hockey or drink. I didn't want to drink. So I played hockey."

By the time he reached adolescence, Ron wasn't bored with his stick, but he was definitely bored with small-town life. "Everybody there grew up the same," he says. "They either put up Sheetrock or they were farmers. It isn't a bad life, I guess, but I just didn't want to do the same thing." Behind Gresch's sleepy façade lies great determination. When Rangers teammate Phil Esposito once accompanied Gresch on a trip home, he said to Ron as they drove around town, "I've got to ask you a very serious question. How did you ever get out of this place?" The answer, of course, is hockey. Encouraged by his family, Gresch joined a farm team in Vancouver and advanced on various junior league teams in Canada. He finally landed on the Rangers squad in 1974. As part of that all-star team, Gresch has distinguished himself by playing fast and furious. Indeed, his energetic playing has occasionally had unfortunate con-

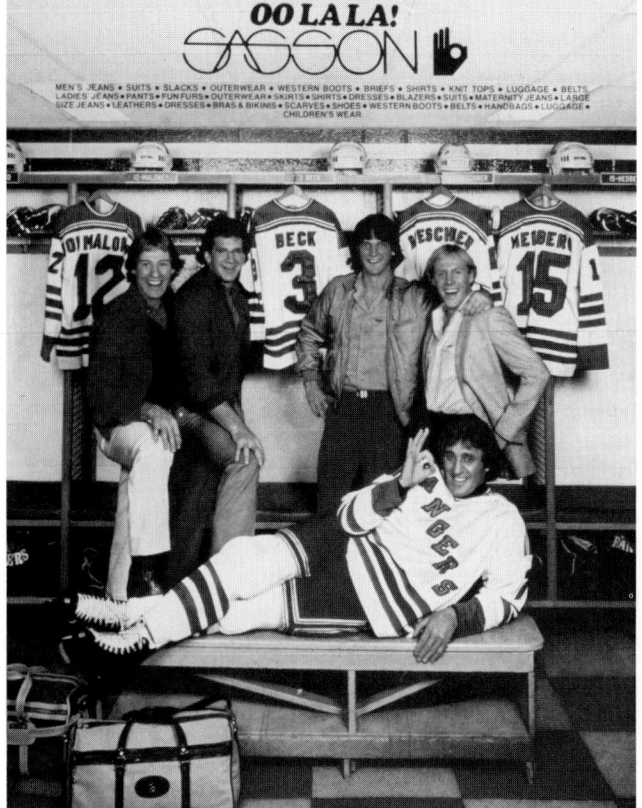

Left: Ron with fashion model Carol Alt.

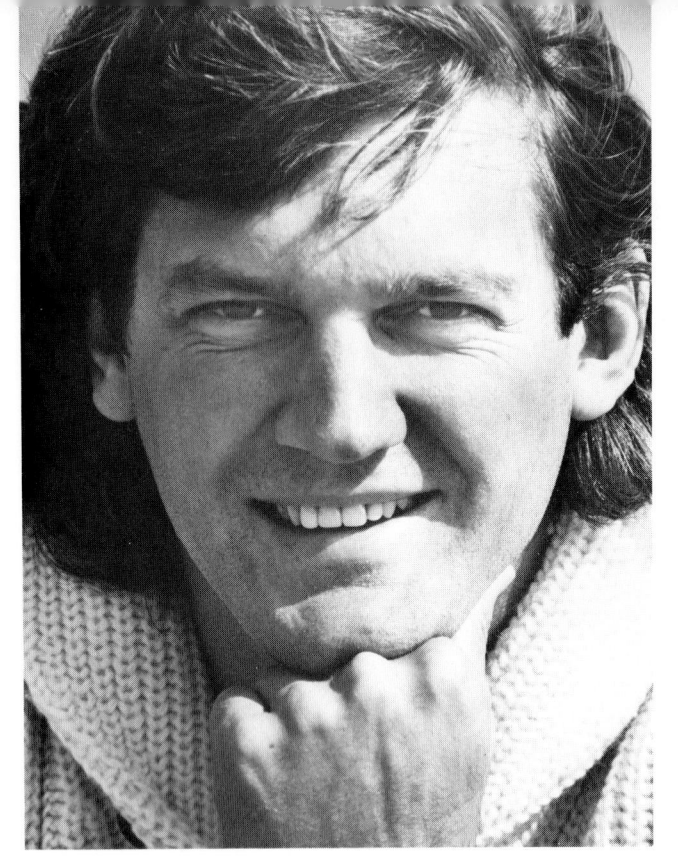

sequences. During a 1981 game, he suffered a serious back injury that kept him sidelined for the rest of that season and part of the 1982–83 season. "The average hockey player used to play seven or eight years," observes Ron. "Now it's more like four or five years. I've been lucky. I've already played eight." But his back injuries cause Gresch to exercise a bit more caution.

Ron Greschner's country-bred charisma is the real thing. He's famous for his generous behavior toward fans who approach him on the street, but Gresch dismisses his friendliness as nothing out of the ordinary. "It makes you feel good," he says matter-of-factly. Gresch's affability was, in fact, partially responsible for the success of the Sasson jeans commercial. "It was a brand-new thing for sports people to be in jeans," he says, "and we had a lot of fun making it. It only took a day, and by the end, we'd had such a good time, we were ready to party." Ironically, the ad became something of an albatross for its participants. Coaches and fans blamed it for an occasional bad showing on the ice. "Whenever you did something wrong, it was blamed on your commercial. It was considered the start of your downfall."

Besides hockey, Ron has another obsession: soap operas. While his teammates go out for a beer in the afternoon, Gresch goes home to catch up with the misadventures of his favorite characters. He first got hooked when he happened to catch *One Life to Live* one afternoon. "There was a woman on the show who was turning on all these guys, and that got me interested. I couldn't believe what was on TV." Ever since, Ron has followed *General Hospital, Ryan's Hope,* and *All My Children.* In fact, his enthusiasm for the soaps led to introductions to some of the principals which in turn led to a cameo appearance on *Ryan's Hope* and an offer from *The Edge of Night.* "I think I'd like to work on soap operas," says Ron. "But it takes a lot of time, and you can't do it unless you do it full-time."

For the moment, though, he is concentrating on recuperating from his injuries and recovering lost time. "I'd always planned on playing until I was thirty-five," he says. "Now, I'll be happy if I can hold out for four or five more years, if my body lets me play. That's all I want. I feel the hourglass is starting to empty out." The only nonhockey sideline that Gresch is entertaining is a New York restaurant that he has opened with several teammates. He still retains a base in his homeland; he has dreams for a cattle ranch in Canada, and he's bought twelve hundred acres there over the last several years.

Ron doesn't envision many more forays into fashion for himself. But he does see one ironic similarity between the worlds of ice and artifice: "What's the average day of a hockey player like? You get up in the morning, you get dressed. You go to the practice rink, get undressed. Put on your equipment, go onto the ice. Skate around for a while, come back off the ice, get undressed, take a shower, put on your clothes again. Go home, come back to the rink for a game, get back into your equipment. All you do all day is get dressed and undressed."

Ron Greschner
Vital & Not So Vital Statistics
Birthdate: December 22, 1954
Height: 6'2"
Weight: 215 lbs.
Hair: Brown
Eyes: Blue
Personal Favorites —
Skates: Lange
Coach: Herb Brooks
Town: New York City
Actors: John Belushi; Gene Wilder
Movie: *Young Frankenstein*
Color: Brown
Car: White Mercedes convertible
TV Shows: *M*A*S*H; The Three Stooges*
Hangouts: Oren and Aretsky, Jim McMullen's, both in New York City
Vacation Spots: Bahamas; Paradise Island; Saskatchewan, Canada
Hobbies: Skiing; water skiing; "I play every sport there is except basketball"; collecting baseball-type caps; playing Intellivision; golf
Drink: Molson's golden ale

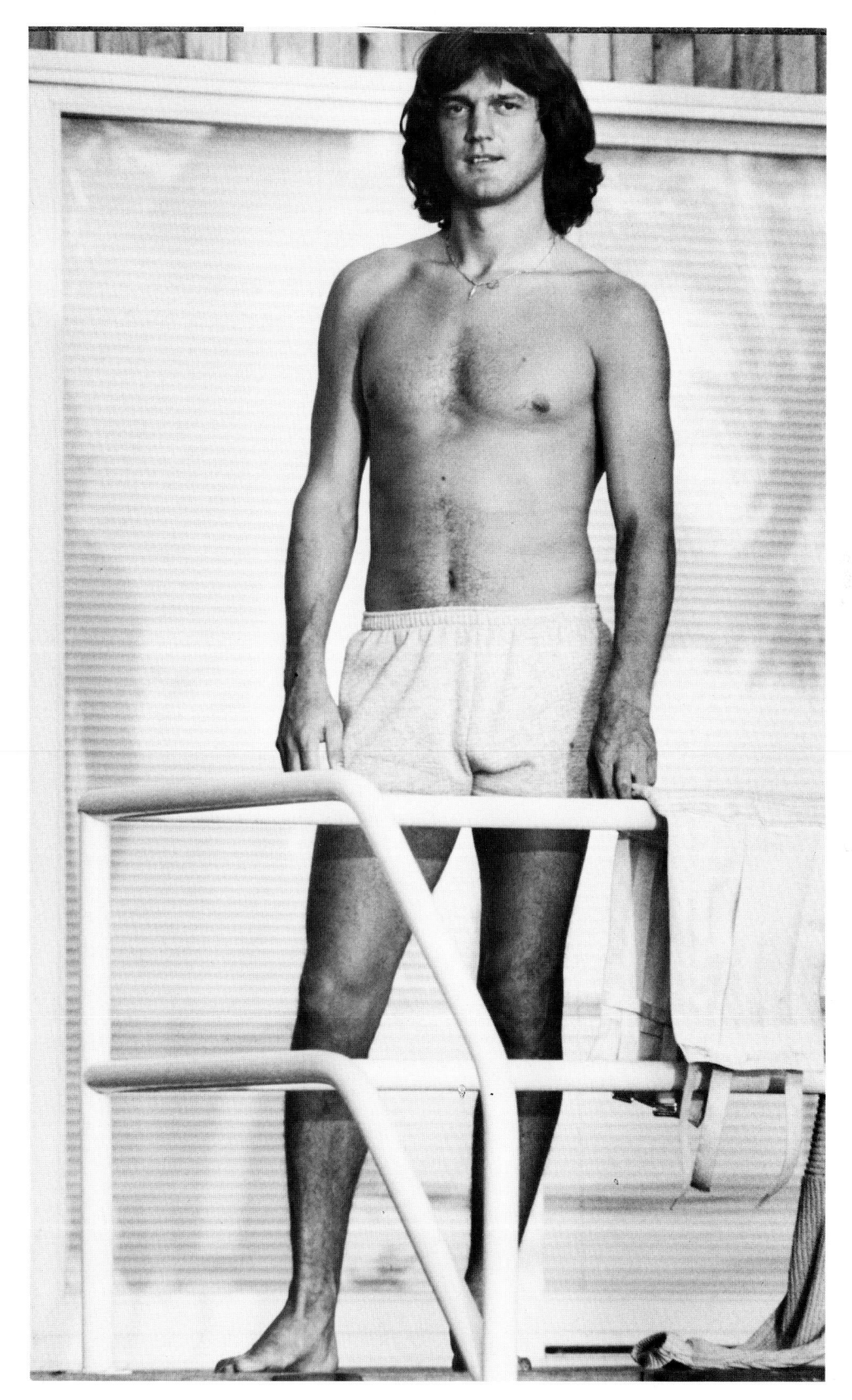

"If I thought hockey was a really violent sport, I wouldn't play. I mean, if you thought you were going out that door and die, you wouldn't walk out the door."

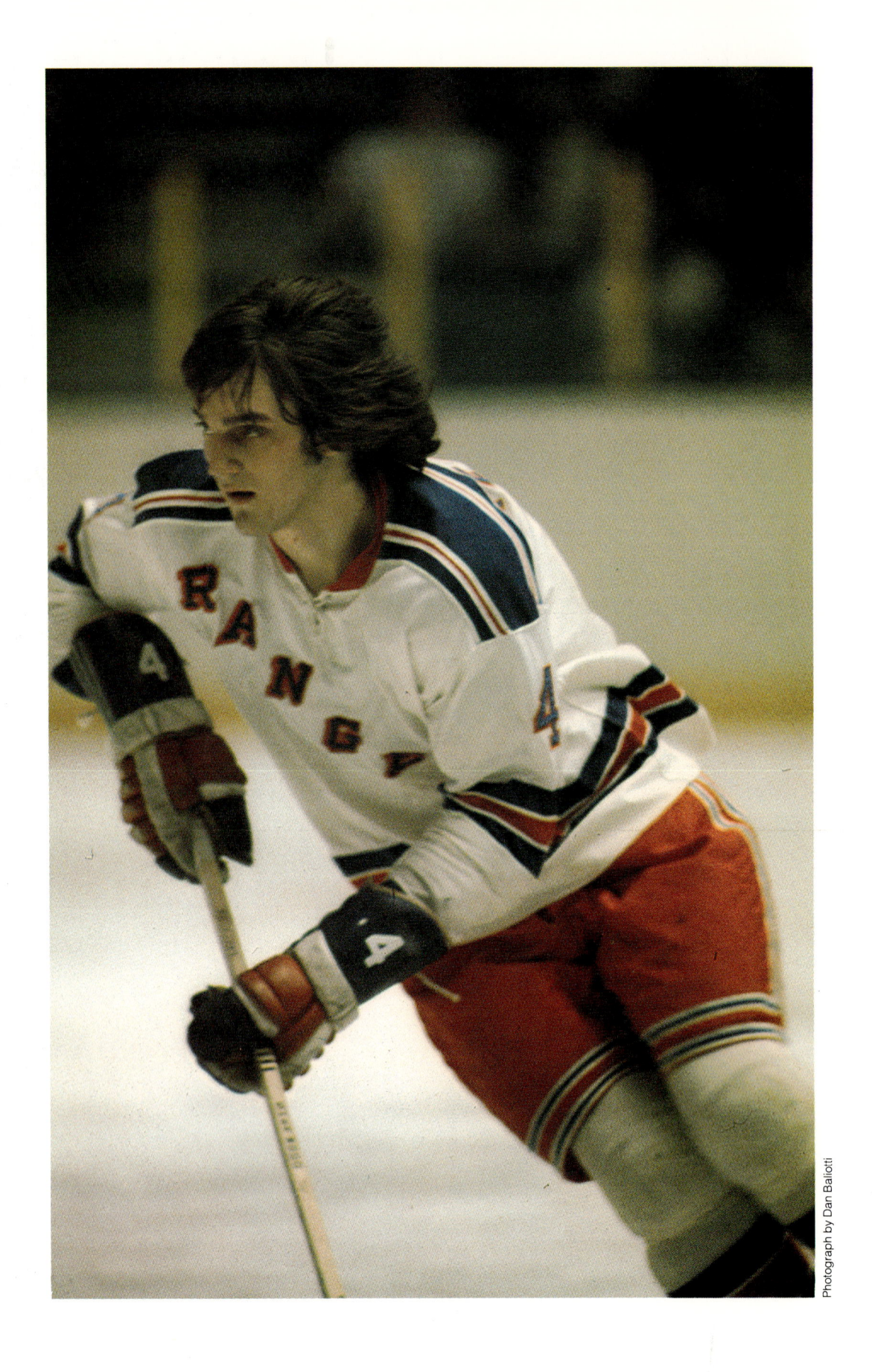

Photograph by Dan Baliotti

'
I love winning.
That's what I like most about hockey. I don't
like to lose – in anything.
'

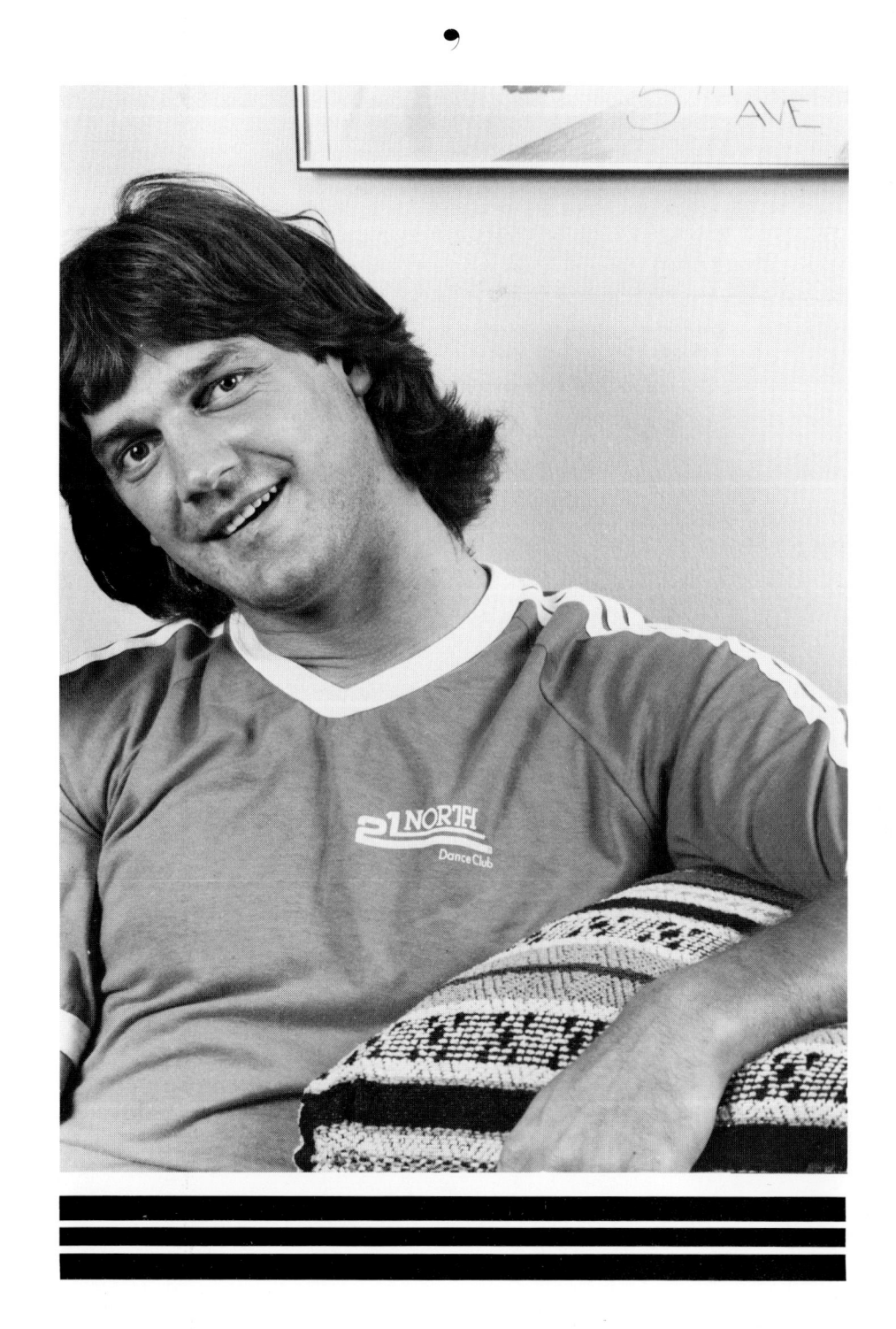

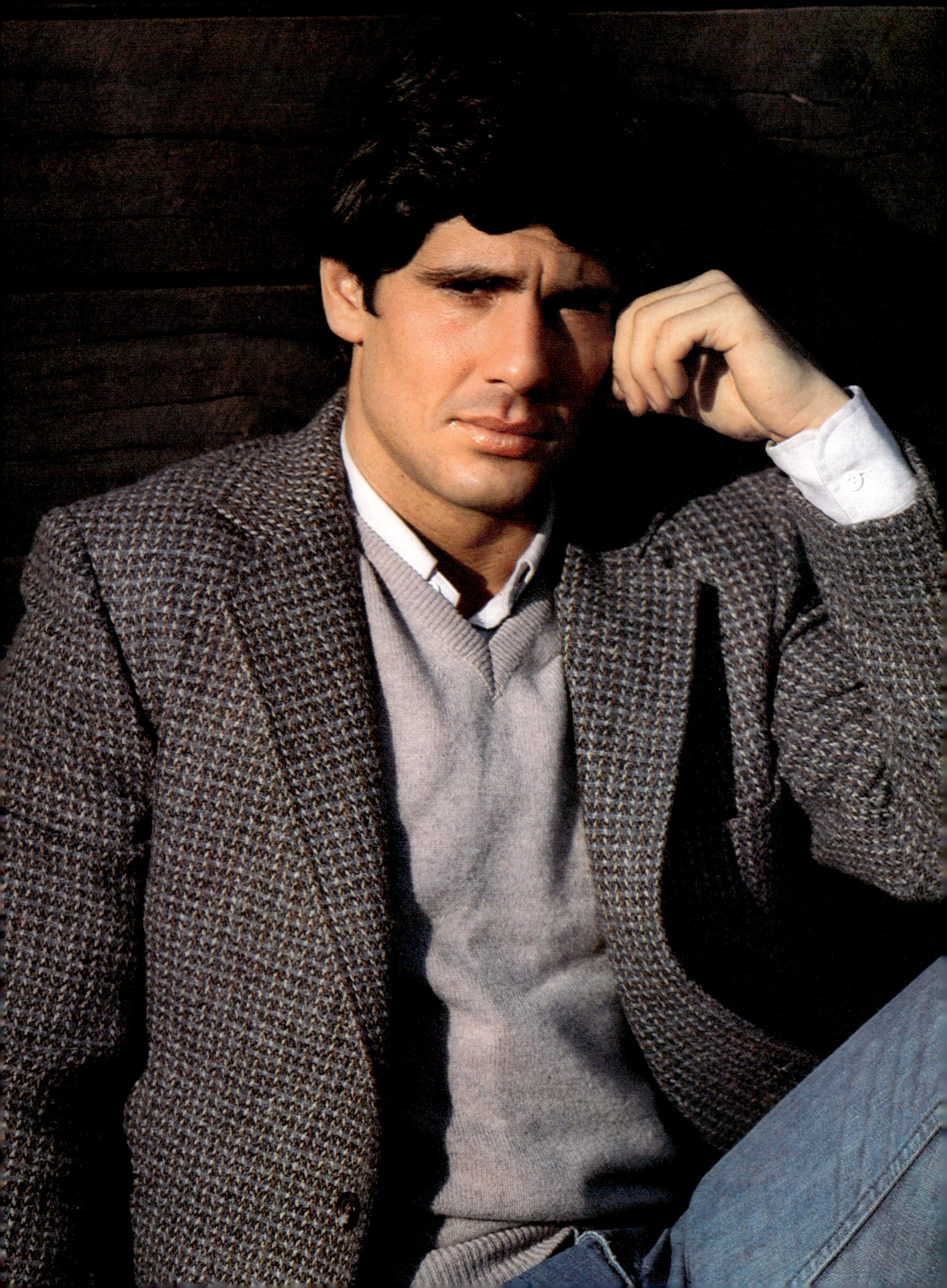

Jason Savas

Jason Savas's signature as a model is a strong, brooding glare into the camera. Not quite a pout and not quite a come-on, it's suspended between sullenness and sensuality — as if Charles Bronson's younger brother were moonlighting as a model. "People *have* told me I look like Charles Bronson," says Jason. "I have a real severe look. It's what I'm known for. It's what I'm most comfortable doing. One of the first photographers I worked with revealed it to me. It's what I learned first, and I fell into it." But Jason insists that his trademark look exists only in front of the camera. "When the shot is over, I'm laughing," he says. "I'm a much more happy-go-lucky guy than those pictures make you think."

Jason is a man of many appearances. Although born in New York City, his dark, strong looks have been represented as Italian, Brazilian, Colombian, Israeli, Greek, and, of course, American. "I'm ethnic, but sort of middle-of-the-road ethnic, so I can do American work or European or whatever," observes Jason. "There aren't a lot of people who look like me, so I can stand out. I can do all sorts of things. Put me in a suit and I pass for a young executive." Put him in a mustache, as a client did on one of Jason's first jobs, and he can pass for Saudi Arabian.

When Jason first tried to enter modeling in 1979, his distinctive looks were, ironically, labeled a liability. "I'm not one of your overnight sensations," he says. "People didn't believe in me at first. It took about eight or nine months before anyone would take a chance on me." Now Jason's versatility has brought him a wealth of work. In addition to television commercials and print work, he has appeared on over 150 book jackets, sometimes in photos, more often in illustrations. "With a costume on for a shot, I can be so many different types of characters," he says. "I can look like a prince from

Photograph by Richard Avedon for Gianni Versace

Gianni Versace

the eighteen hundreds, or a cowboy. It's fun to do book covers because it's a change and it involves a bit of acting."

The real Jason Savas is "a frustrated athlete," he says. Indeed, from Jason's point of view, modeling is now peopled with similarly frustrated jocks. "Nearly all of the guys have played sports," he notes, "but most of us weren't good enough to make the pros. We can't make a living playing sports, even if we want to. But it still means a lot to us. We've got good bodies, we're in shape, we're healthy. And we follow sports. There are a lot of healthy bodies getting into modeling." Although he excelled at wrestling and judo, Jason always wanted to be a pro football or baseball player. He still considers winning his two New York City wrestling championships the most memorable moments of his life. And as a high school athlete, Jason insisted that his parents paint his bedroom walls silver and black — the team colors of his favorite squad, the Oakland Raiders. "Lifetime jock, that's my occupation," says Jason.

The son of a doctor and the second-oldest child in a Greek family of eight, Jason began modeling not long after graduation from New York's City College, where he earned a degree in physical education. While recuperating from an operation, Jason worked as a waiter at the Carlyle Hotel, where he served such celebrities as Warren Beatty, Jack Lemmon, and Raquel Welch. So many patrons of the restaurant asked him if he was a model that he decided to try the profession. Despite the frequent rejection accorded an ethnic type, Jason persisted. "Rejection never bothered me," he says. "I've got more important things to think about."

With his financial success, Jason has realized one of his athletic dreams. He has transformed the twelve acres of his family's home in New Jersey into his own mini sports complex. He has built a tennis court, installed a batting cage with a pitching machine, set up basketball, volleyball, handball, and badminton courts, and laid out a dirt trail for his four dirt bikes. There's also a pond, and, in his living quarters in the basement, a Universal weight machine and wrestling mat. "I put a nice chunk of money into this," says Jason, who lives alone during the week in a spacious eight-room apartment on Manhattan's Upper West Side. "I always wanted to have all the facilities in my backyard to play whenever I want." In New Jersey, Jason's room is littered with baseball mitts, tennis balls, tennis racquets, lacrosse equipment, Frisbees, boomerangs, camping gear, roller skates, ice skates, and skis. "I like to work hard in the city and then bring my friends out here and play ball,

> I'll always be in shape.
> It doesn't have
> anything to do with the business.
> It's just a part of me.
> If I didn't work out,
> I wouldn't be happy. I'd be
> frustrated.

or bring girlfriends and just take it easy and lie in the sun."

Since Jason is an accomplished, enthusiastic cook, the kitchen is almost as well stocked as the playing fields. "I've got a great kitchen," he says. "Two stoves, two sinks, a ten-foot eating table that will seat twenty people, and a big stainless-steel counter. I like to experiment with cooking and take wild recipes out of books." For the immediate future, Jason intends to continue modeling as long as possible. He also has aspirations to write — fiction, short pieces, screenplays — but he hesitates to discuss those plans. "I don't like to talk about anything until I do it," he says. "I'm a *doer.* I do things and then let people know who I am."

Jason Savas
Vital & Not So Vital Statistics
Birthdate: November 21, 1954
Height: 5'11½"
Weight: 165 lbs.
Hair: Brown
Eyes: Brown

Personal Favorites —
Drink: Milk
Breakfast: Blueberry pancakes
Football Team: Oakland Raiders
Music: Rock and roll: Rolling Stones; Pink Floyd
Color: Silver
Actors: Jack Nicholson; Charles Bronson; Clint Eastwood
Movie: *Apocalypse Now*
Hobbies: Softball; tennis; dirt bikes; writing
Vacation Spot: Negril Beach, Jamaica
Town: East Hampton, New York
Hangouts: Teacher's, Marvin Gardens, Pumpkin Eater, all in New York City
Athletes: Willie Mays; Al Kaline; Carl Yastrzemski
Hero: Pete Rose
Agency: Wilhelmina, New York City

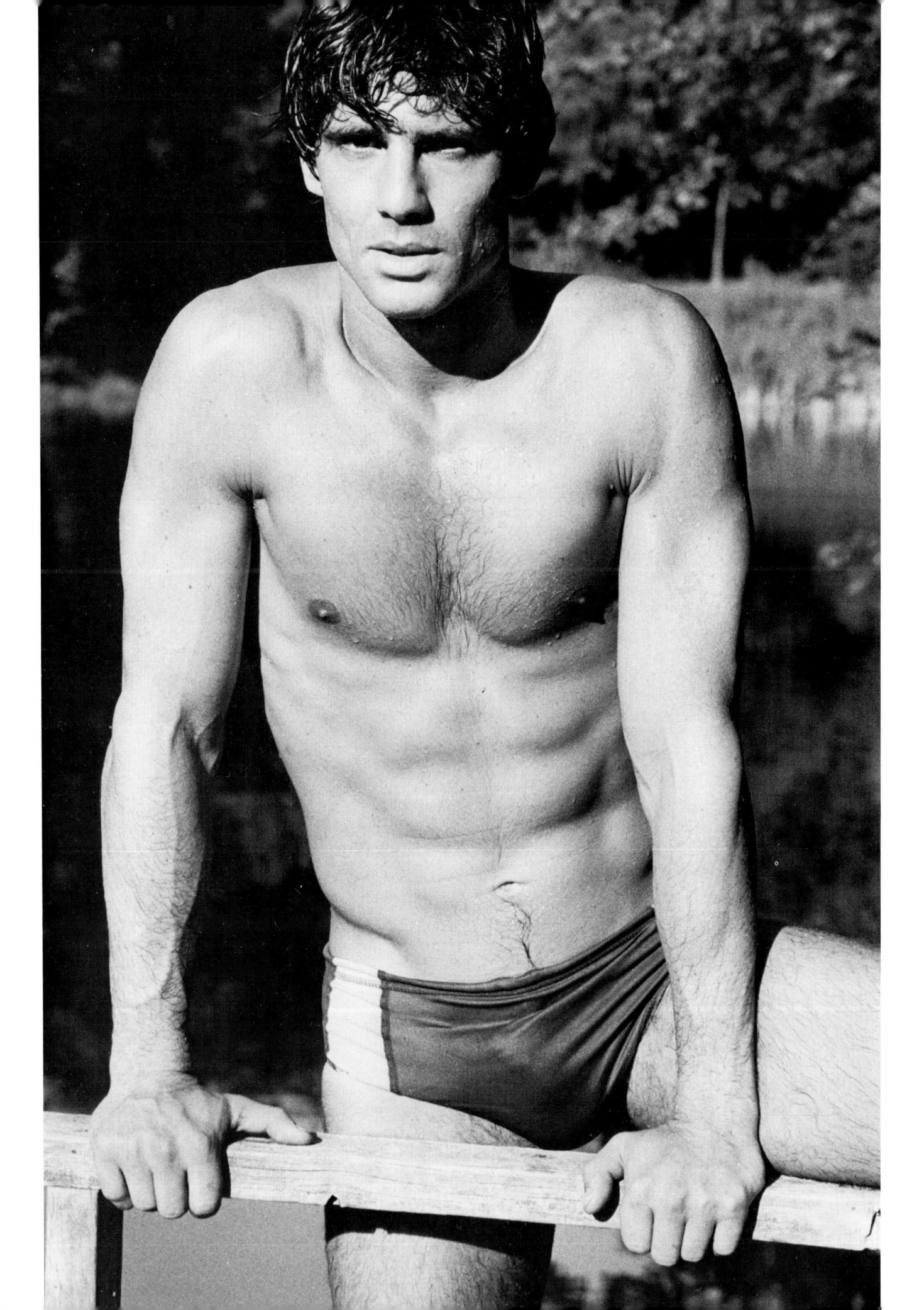

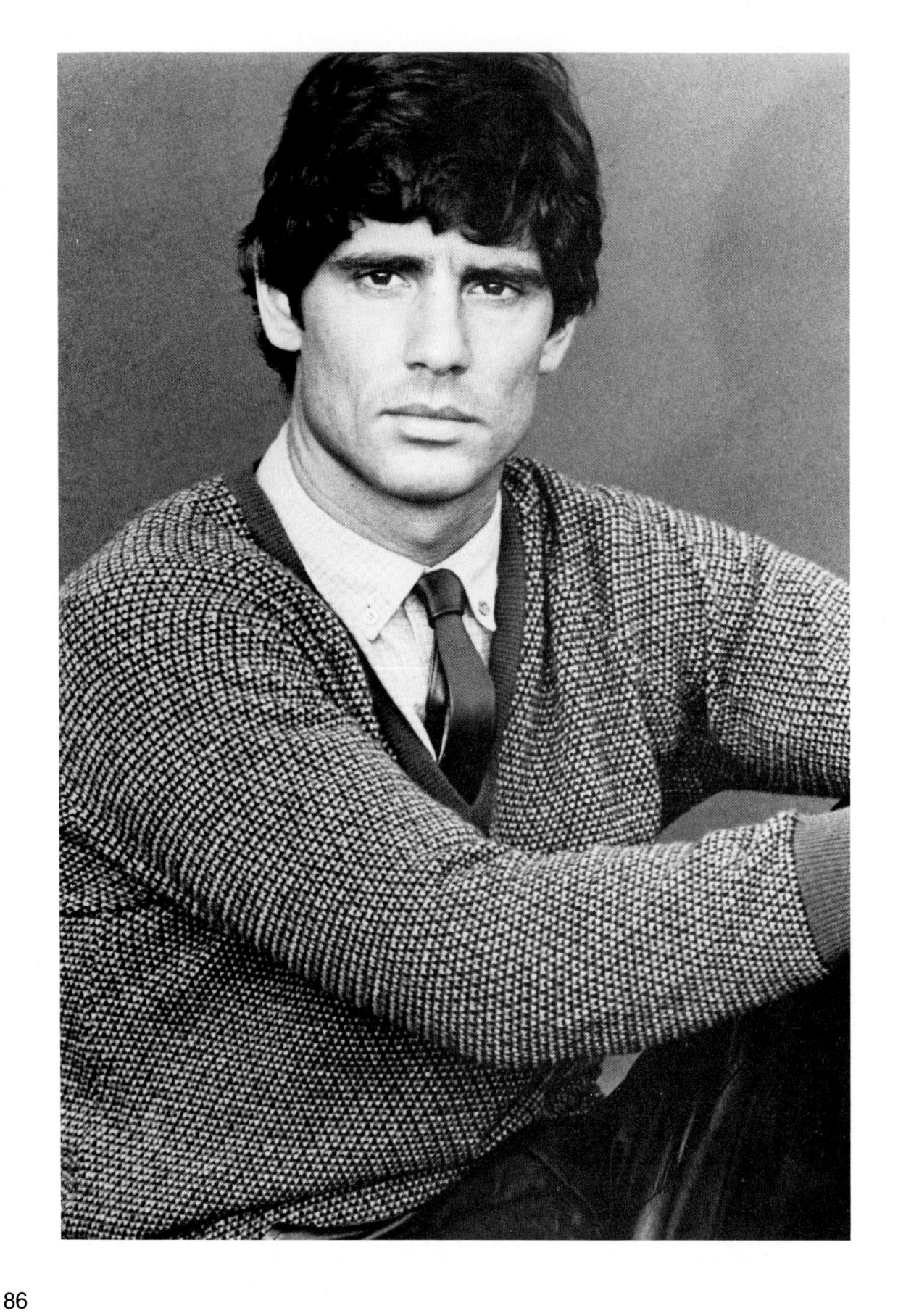

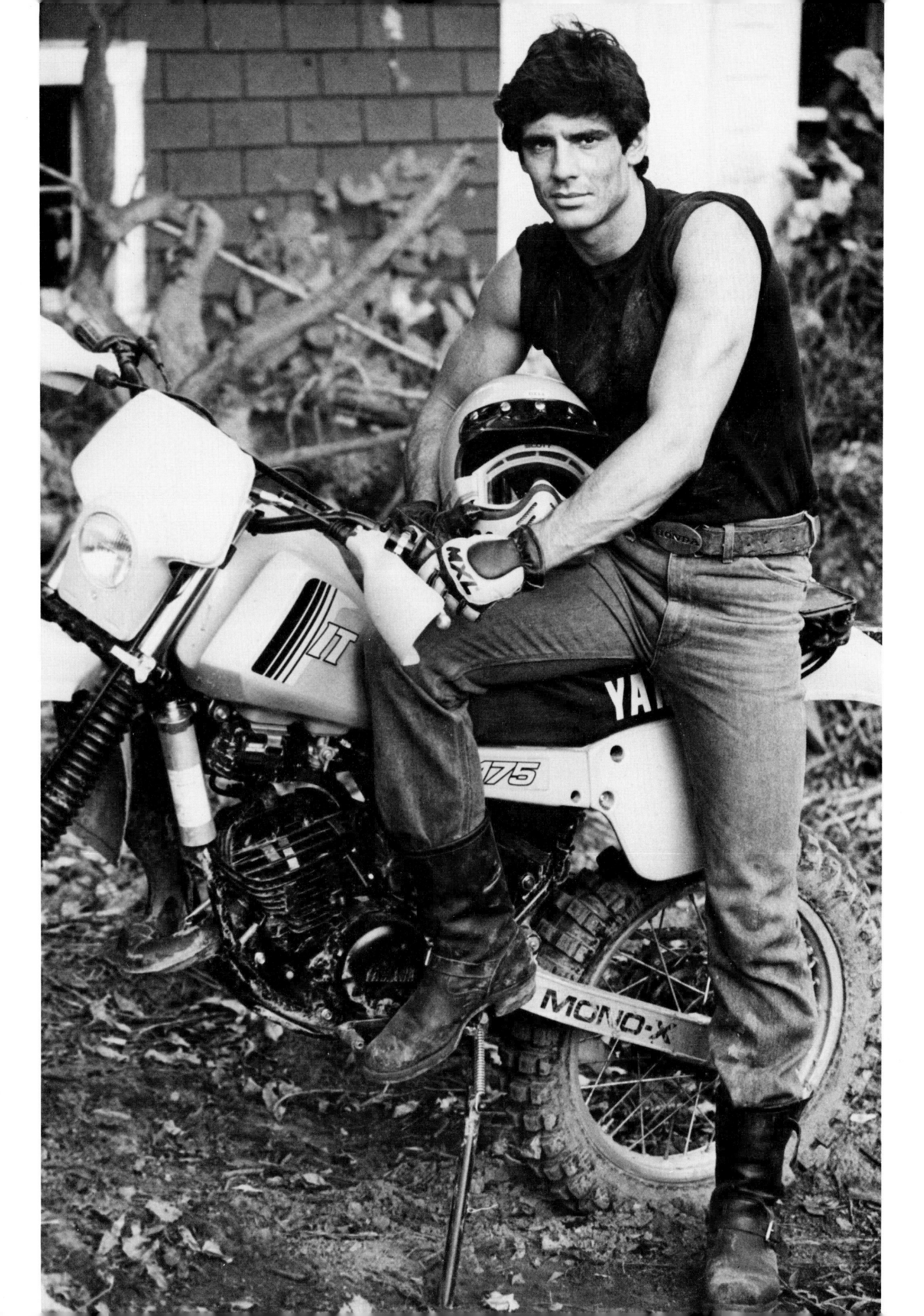

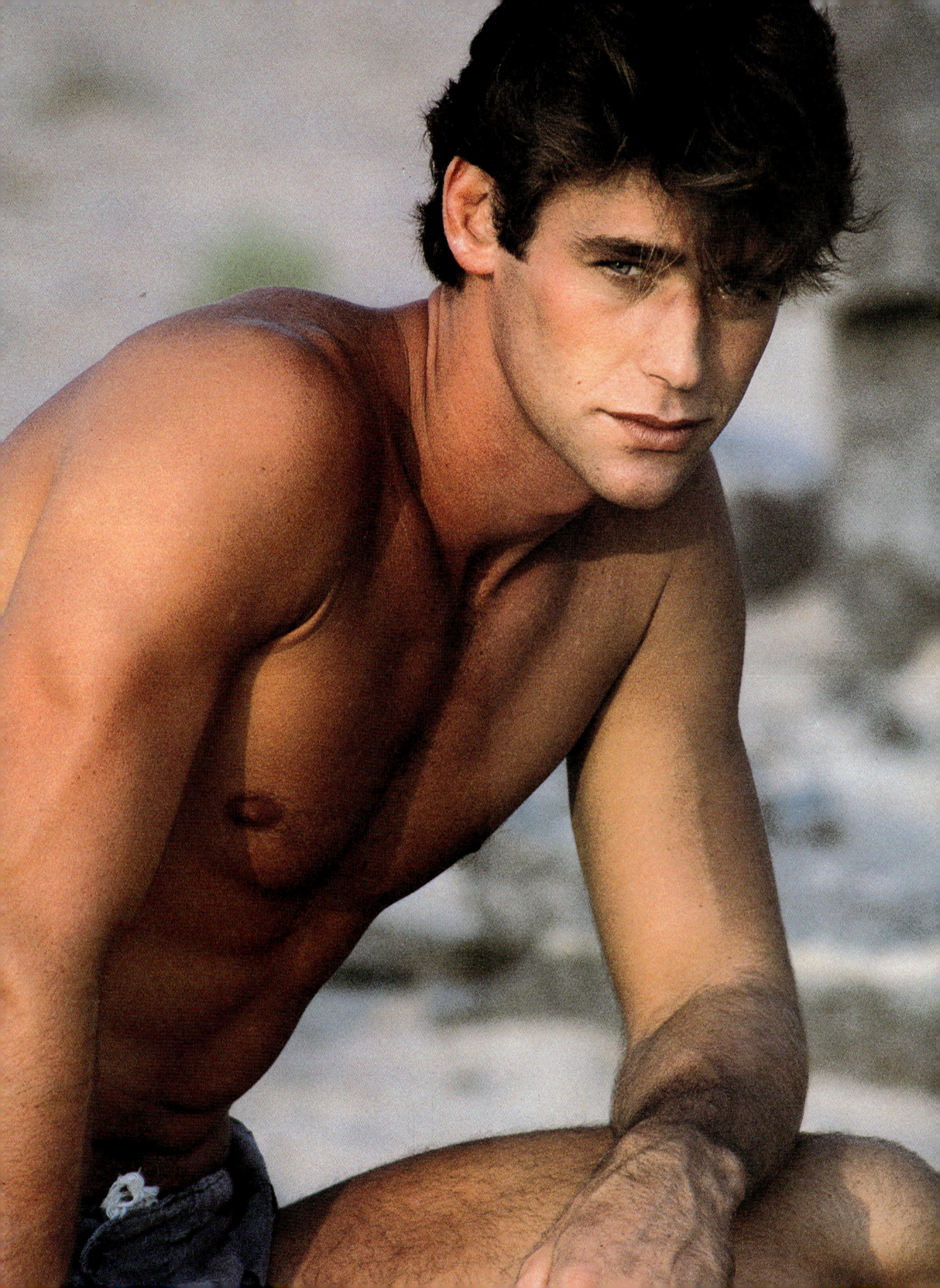

Todd Irvin

Todd Irvin's roots are pure Americana. The son of a business executive and an interior decorator, Todd grew up in Chagrin Falls, Ohio, a picturesque small town that epitomizes the country's heartland. "Chagrin Falls has a real Huck Finn aura," says Todd. "There *is* a falls running through it, and it's small, so there's a real community. I've known all my friends there since age one."

Todd's all-American looks have taken him far away from Chagrin Falls, of course. Ironically, his handsomeness was first appreciated not in this country but by fashion photographers in Europe. A *magna cum laude* graduate of Duke University, with a bad case of wanderlust, Todd was traveling through Europe when he fell into modeling in 1978. In Paris, Todd was supposed to stay with a family friend, and he went to pick up the apartment keys at a modeling agency for which his friend worked. "I arrived in hiking boots with a backpack and a beard," Todd says, "and I walked into this nice low-lit place with all these gorgeous girls walking around." The agency suggested that Todd sign up, and he did—only to regret the decision immediately. A stranger in a strange land and profession, he felt disoriented and disenchanted. "I'd go through these moments when I just couldn't do what the photographer wanted," recalls Todd. Out of that confusion and awkwardness evolved his now top-dollar trademark: a cosmopolitan blasé gaze *away* from the camera, a semibored look punctuated by piercing blue eyes and pouting lower lip. "That was just the intense defiance I felt when I started getting work in Europe," says Todd. "It was a way to relate to the camera because I couldn't get into it and say, 'Oh, these are beautiful clothes.' " Todd defends his unconventional approach as honest. "I'm very camera-shy, so I'm either rebelling or laughing at it as a way to get by." And that look puts him in a unique, much sought after position. "My whole image is that of the *anti-model*. Let's face it, everybody cultivates an image. When I first started, I almost looked spiteful, insulting, sarcastic about what I was doing." But as his career has skyrocketed, Todd's world-

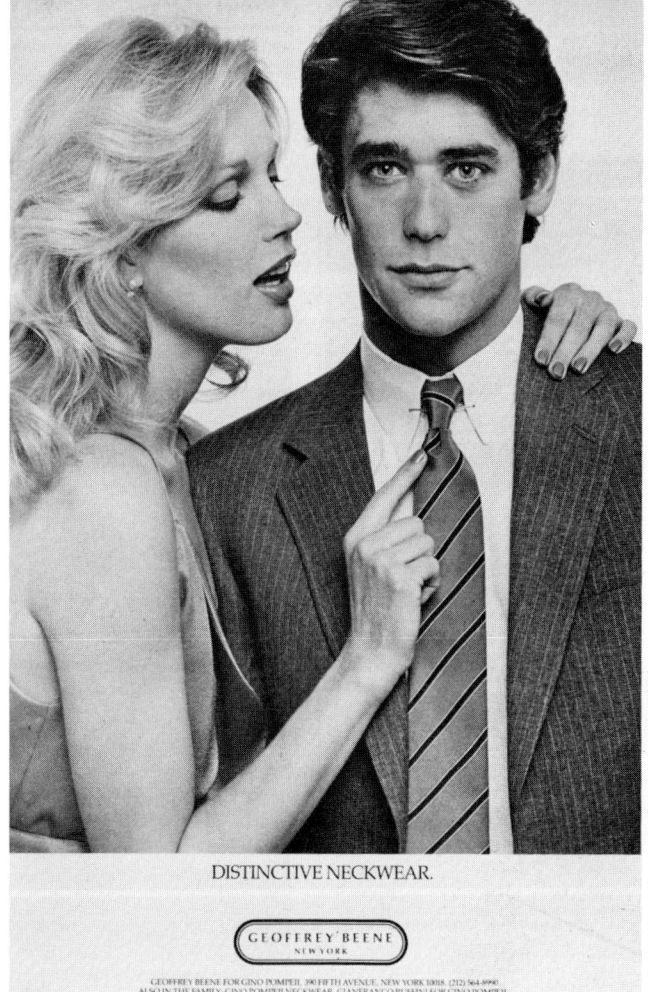

DISTINCTIVE NECKWEAR.

GEOFFREY BEENE
NEW YORK

Photograph & Design: Sisyphus Advertising

weary expression has softened a bit. "It's been toned down," observes Todd. "I've been a little homogenized, made more middle-of-the-road."

After two years in Paris, Todd's Continental success caught the attention of American agencies. When he returned to Chagrin Falls for Christmas one year, he received a call from Zoli, a New York agency. Recalls Todd, "A woman asked, 'How would you like to go down to Key West on New Year's Day and do something for Calvin Klein and Bruce Weber?' I said, 'Great,' but I didn't know who Calvin Klein and Bruce Weber were at the time."

Working in America proved quite a different experience, and, as an amateur anthropologist, the differences fascinated Todd. "In Europe, fashion has a nice identity or status as one of the sister arts. Fashion has permeated the culture in a lot of ways, and therefore Europeans are more comfortable about it. It's more relaxed, more casual. Here, fashion is more of a business. People are more serious and more professional about it. There's a greater grandeur in Europe and no male hang-ups about working as a model."

Todd's characteristically cavalier look belies his serious, analytical nature. A constant student of psychology, he expects to enter the field eventually. "Even in Paris, I was pursuing the psych thing," he says. "I was working at a crisis center for English-speaking people in Paris. It was a telephone service called S.O.S." Todd would like to combine his interest in movies with his education in psychology—perhaps by developing the role and use of film in psychiatric intervention techniques.

Personable and energetic, Todd says he is "far from identifying directly with my image in front of the camera." Although he lives in the Chelsea section of New York City, Todd's home away from home is his island retreat in northern Ontario. "I've traveled a lot of places, but that is really one of the most beautiful I've ever seen. I restore my sanity there. It's just rock, pines and a lot of water."

In an important way, Todd's print persona and his off-camera self coincide. He views modeling with the sort of detachment one would expect of the fellow in his pictures. "You've *got* to laugh at it a little," says Todd. "Any guy who believes all the glamor stuff and believes in the game has got a lot to learn. Otherwise, you end up like that actor who played Superman on television, the one who believed his image and tried to fly. You can end up in a lot of trouble."

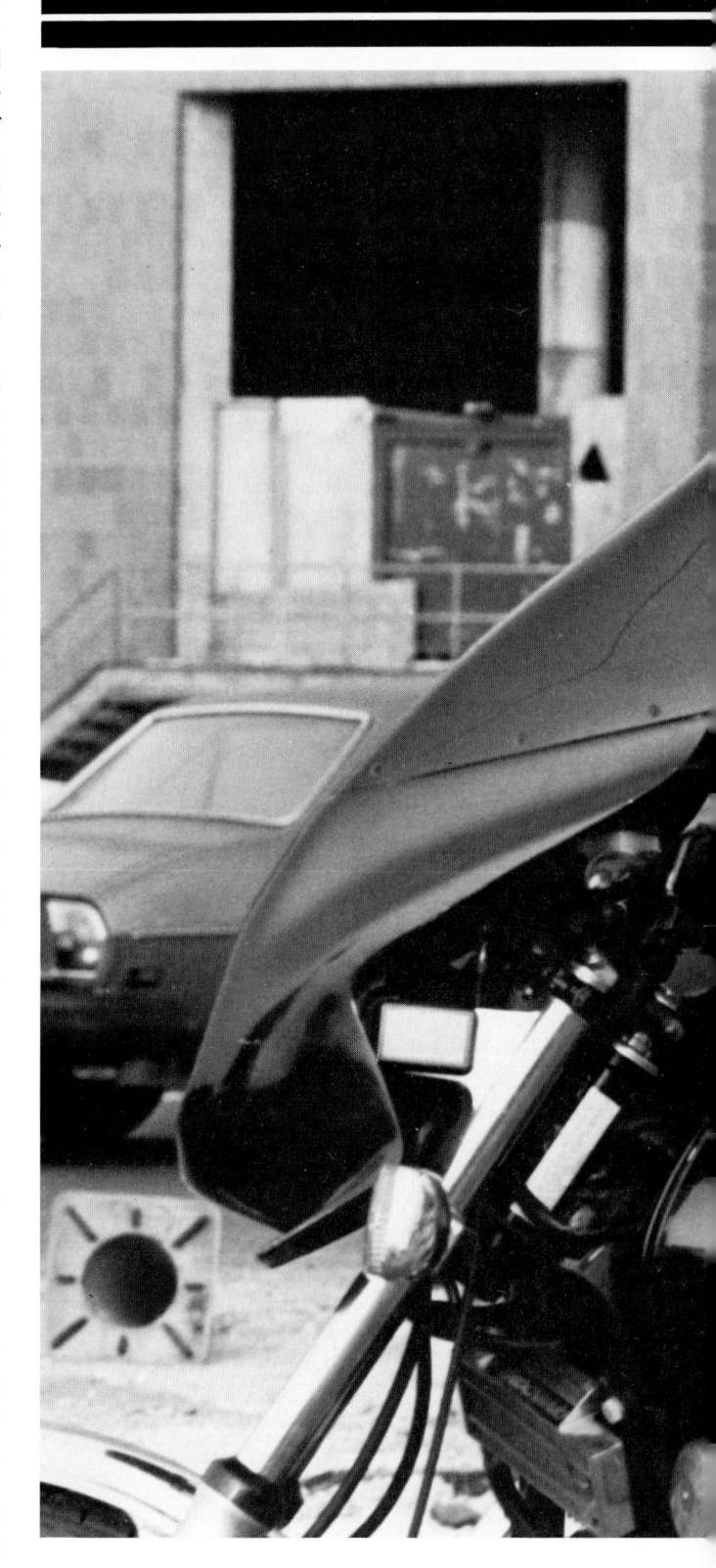

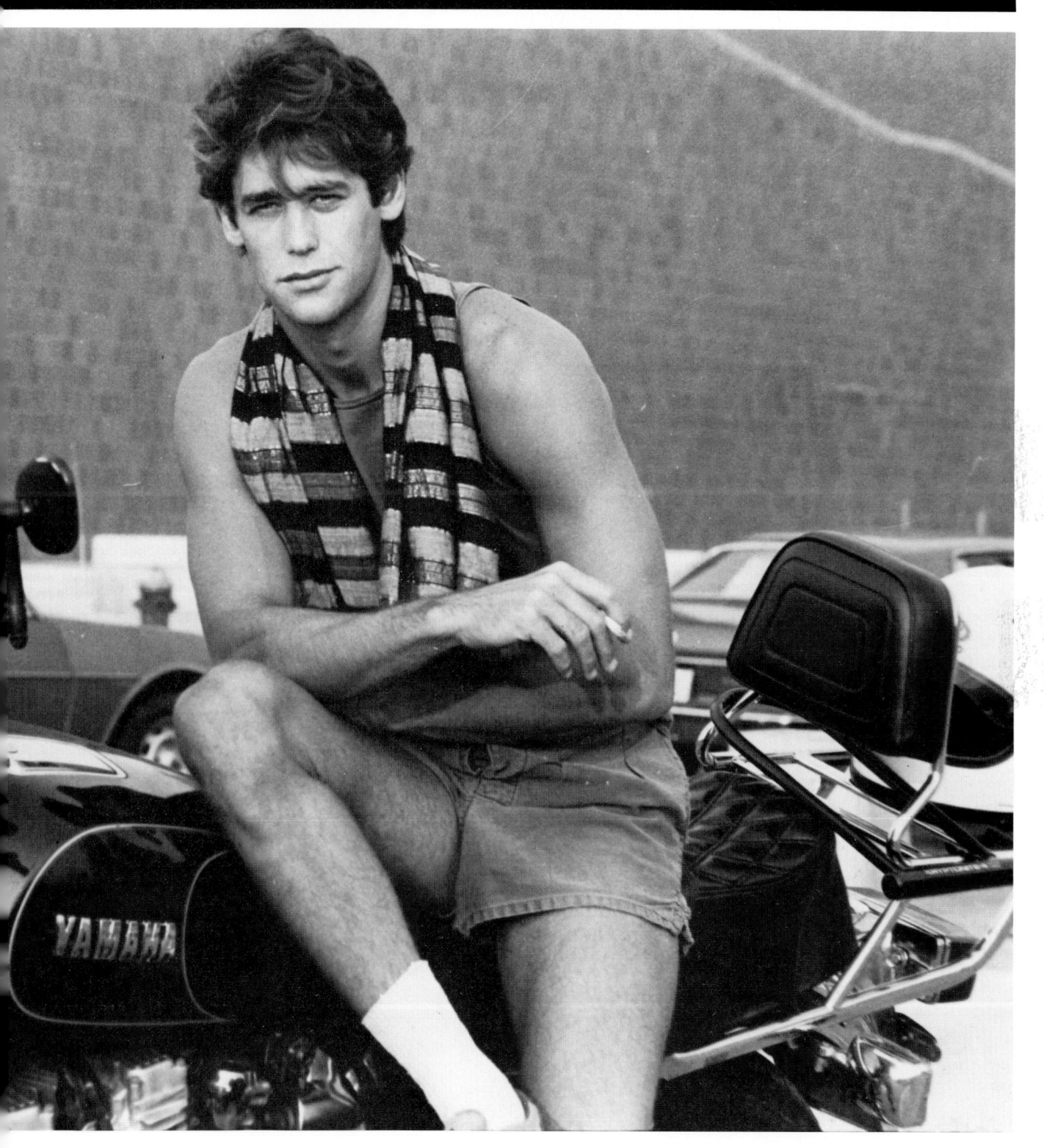

"I considered traveling to Europe part of my personal development. I was getting a little distance on my own culture. The foreign experience gets you to crystalize what your own experience is about."

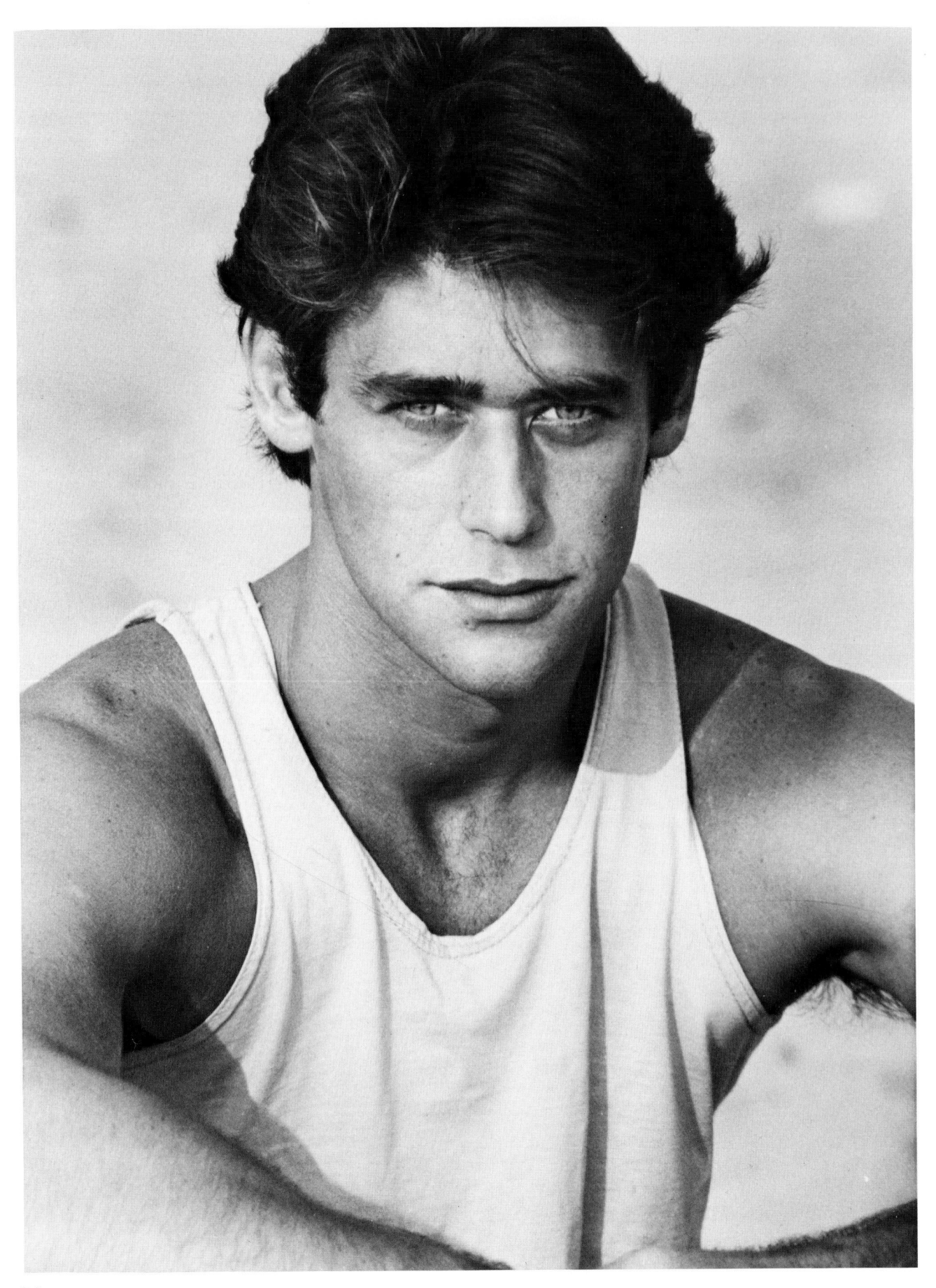

> I think the
> male population in general —
> and specifically
> men who are considered
> good-looking — want
> to play that element
> down or
> not draw
> attention to it.
> With me, there's a real
> fear of being
> typecast as a Don Juan
> or Joe Stud.
> I always felt a need
> to dress down.

Todd Irvin

Vital & Not So Vital Statistics
Birthdate: August 31, 1956
Height: 6′1½″
Weight: 180 lbs.
Hair: Brown
Eyes: Blue

Personal Favorites —
Color: Georgian Bay-blue
Vacation Spot: Point Au Baril, Ontario
After-shave: Cibel
Books: *The Magus,* by John Fowles; *Despair,* by Vladimir Nabokov
Cartoon: *Looney Tunes*
Actor: Ronald Reagan
Movies: *Last Tango in Paris; Cool Hand Luke; Carnal Knowledge; The Wizard of Oz*
Town: Chagrin Falls, Ohio
Snack: Snickers Bars
Drink: Labat's Blue Beer
Music: Jazz-blues; country western
Hobbies: Sketching; antique collecting; breeding dogs
Sports: Canoeing; sailing; windsurfing; motorcycling; skiing
Taste in Women: "Presence with beauty"
Hangouts: The Ojibway Hotel, Katmandu; La Coupole, Paris; Scotty's Bar, New York City
Ambition: "People used to ask me what I wanted to do and I'd tell them I wanted to gather coconuts. Now I want to own the coconut tree."
Agency: Zoli, New York City

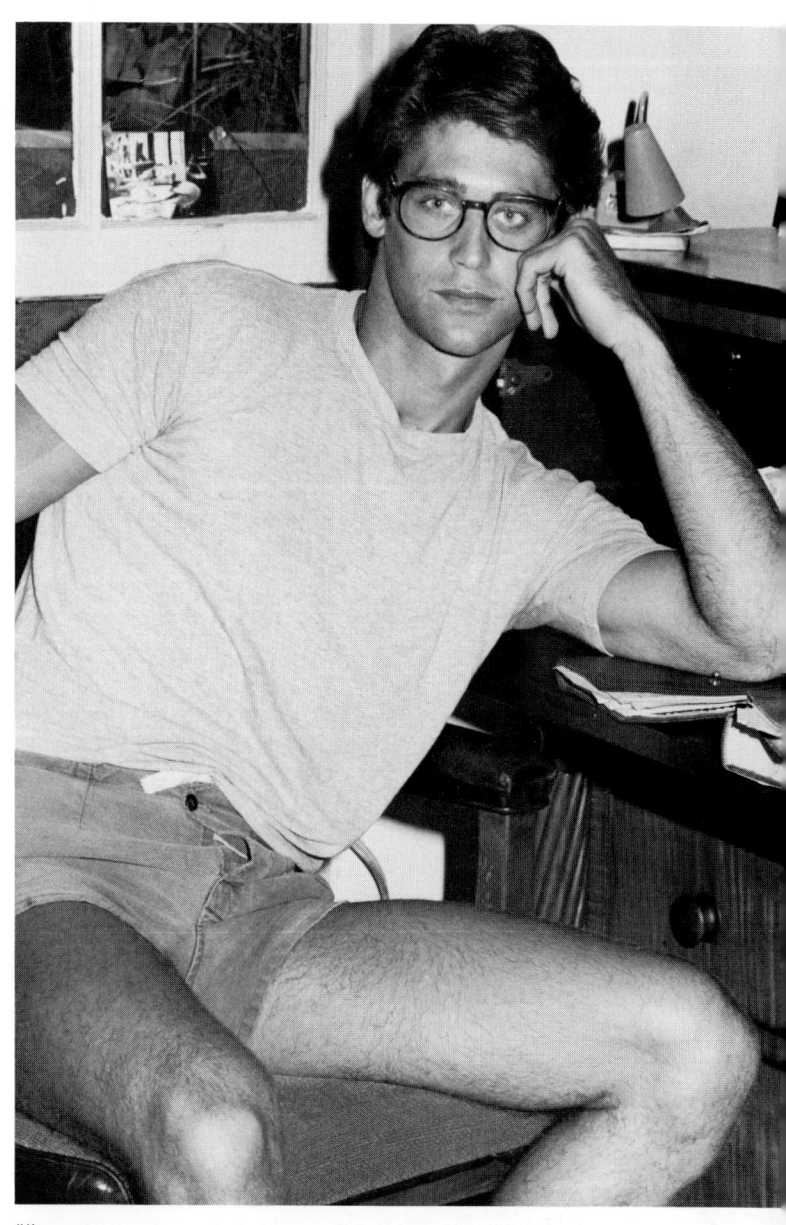

"I'm not an extroverted person. Someone who is basically shy can often be interpreted as being cocky or conceited."

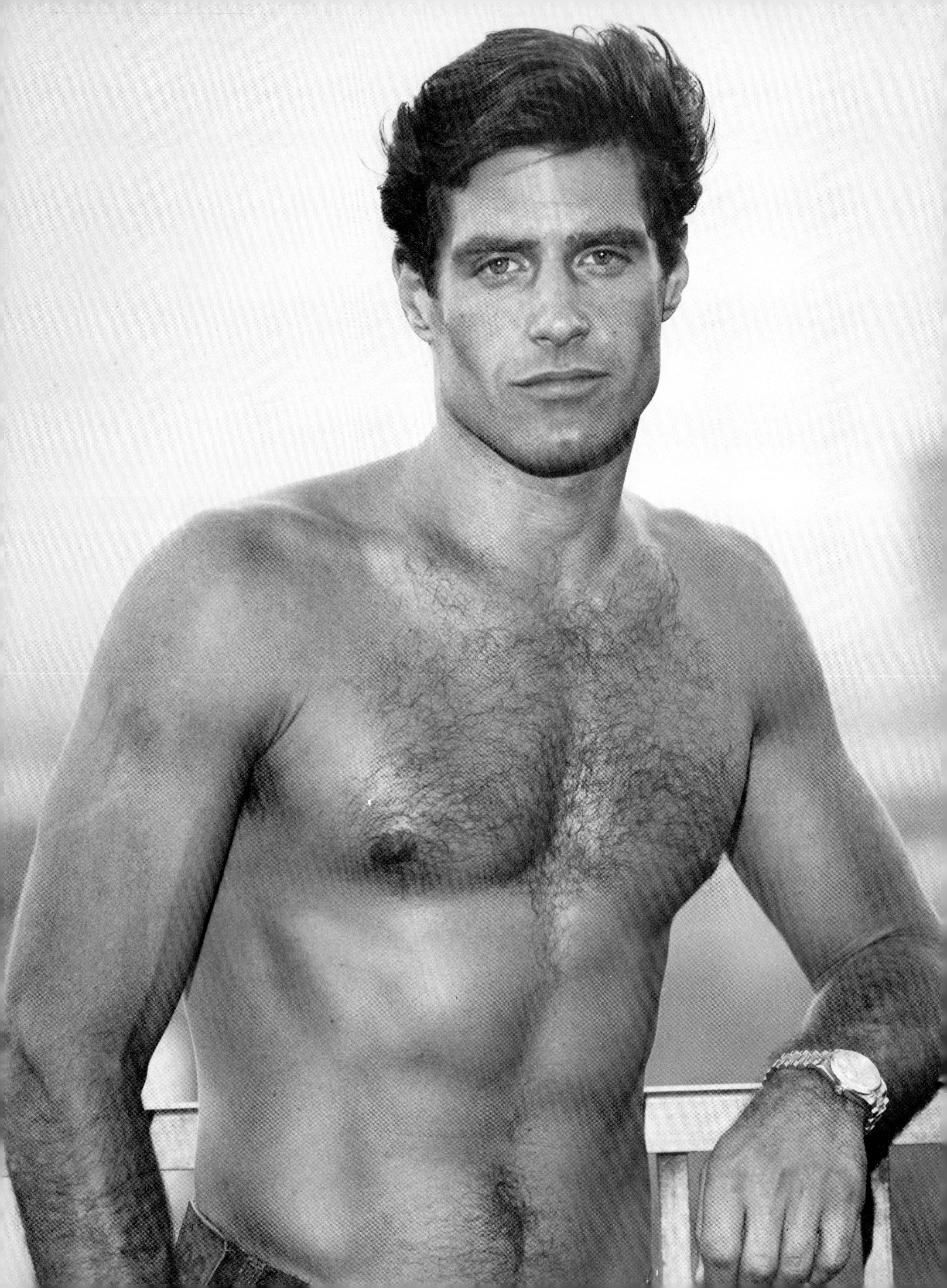

Scott Webster

Scott Webster likes the view from the top — and he has a penthouse to prove it. Scott lives in a duplex overlooking Central Park in New York City. The brass-and-marble co-op is designed to suit Scott's high style. There's a sauna in one of the four bathrooms, a giant television screen in the "media" room, and a refrigerator in the master bedroom so Scott needn't trek downstairs to the kitchen for one of his beloved light beers. His duplex is awash in luxury, and, says Scott, "money seems to be the root of what drives me. I came to New York to make money and over the past three years, I've averaged over two hundred thousand dollars a year in modeling. I make money and I know how to invest it. It takes more than good looks to be a model. If you think models are dumb, just look at my bank account."

As one of the industry's undisputed superstars, Scott has a unique trademark: a defiant, I-dare-you staredown with the camera. In his photos, he looks at once sophisticated and self-involved, a touch of class mixed with a touch of evil. Scott doesn't mind the malevolent undercurrent of his photographs. "I've never been a good boy," he says. "There's some devil in me, and it comes out." Scott describes his look as "American elegance, the gentleman off the field" and his chiseled features as "classical." According to Scott, "Not many people have it. You know — high bones, cut face, strong jaw. In modeling, there's always this year's trendy look, whether it's French or Italian or whatever. But my classic American look is going to be around forever."

Scott plots his career with the cool, bottom-line pragmatism of a businessman — which is, in fact, his chosen profession. A seasoned buyer of real estate, Scott owns property in Illinois, Florida, and New York, and he's made "over seven figures" in real estate deals. Scott has consciously used modeling as "a means to an end." As he observes, "Modeling generates cash flow and it lets me pursue my business deals." Among Scott's best buddies are the lawyers and stockbrokers who advise him on financial matters.

Business inadvertently prompted Scott to start modeling. Scott grew up in the well-to-do suburb of Lake Forest, Illinois, and while studying business administration at Northern Illinois University, he began to speculate in the commodities market. After five months and some ill-advised trades, he had lost twenty thousand dollars. To repay his debts, he began modeling with Victor Skrebneski in Chicago, then moved east when top bookings beckoned.

While Scott looks like one of the elite in front of the camera, he quickly turns into one of the boys at home, particularly when he's watching Monday night football. He answers his phone with a boisterous "Harry's Bar and Grill," and he often has a beer handy. He regularly enjoys nights on the town in fancy restaurants with his informal fraternity of friends. A rabble-rouser in an expensive suit, Scott insists, "We get wild in *good* places, not cheap joints."

If there's one thing that rubs Scott the wrong way, it's the common — and, he says, mistaken — perception that models are vain. According to Scott, "If I walk up to a mirror after working my ass off and look at myself lean and strong with no shirt on and say, 'Man, I look good,' what's wrong with that?" he asks. Ever the entrepreneur, Scott says, "It's my *business* to look good."

How does Scott achieve the distinctive poses that have made him so much in demand? "If they want a sexy look, I look into the lens and think of something that turns me on. I mean, I can get *so* into it, it's ridiculous. When you look into a model's eye, you just let her get into your heart. There can be fifty other people around you, pedestrians on the street, but you don't even see them. When you don't see anything but the thoughts in your head, then you're working. You're a pro."

Scott has his own theory about his astounding success: he sees himself as a convincing emblem of privilege. "I believe in success. It would take most corporate executives ten years or more before they could enter the income bracket I'm in. When *I* stand in front of a Rolls-Royce, people know Scott Webster can own a Rolls-Royce. When I'm in the car in a tuxedo with a beautiful woman, and I take the wheel, the camera knows I belong there. That's the difference. It's why I'm successful. When you've risen to the top, you can comfortably say what you do for a living."

Scott Dayton Webster

Vital & Not So Vital Statistics
Birthdate: April 25, 1955
Height: 6'
Weight: 165 lbs.
Hair: Light brown
Eyes: Blue

Personal Favorites —
Car: Rolls-Royce Corniche
TV Show: *60 Minutes*
Time of Day: Night
Vacation Spot: Bermuda
Metal: Gold
Town: Manhattan
Actor: Clint Eastwood
Movies: *Dirty Harry; The Good, the Bad, and the Ugly*
Actress: Marilyn Monroe
Magazines: *Forbes; Money; Playboy*
Hobbies: Tennis; squash; golf; commercial speculation
Cologne: Hermès
Toothpaste: Ultra Brite
Dress Style: "I wear grubby clothes like Lee jeans and a shirt or I wear a seven-hundred-dollar suit. It's one or the other. I always wear my gold Rolex."
Restaurants: Palm, Four Seasons, La Cantina, all in New York City
Agency: Ford, New York City

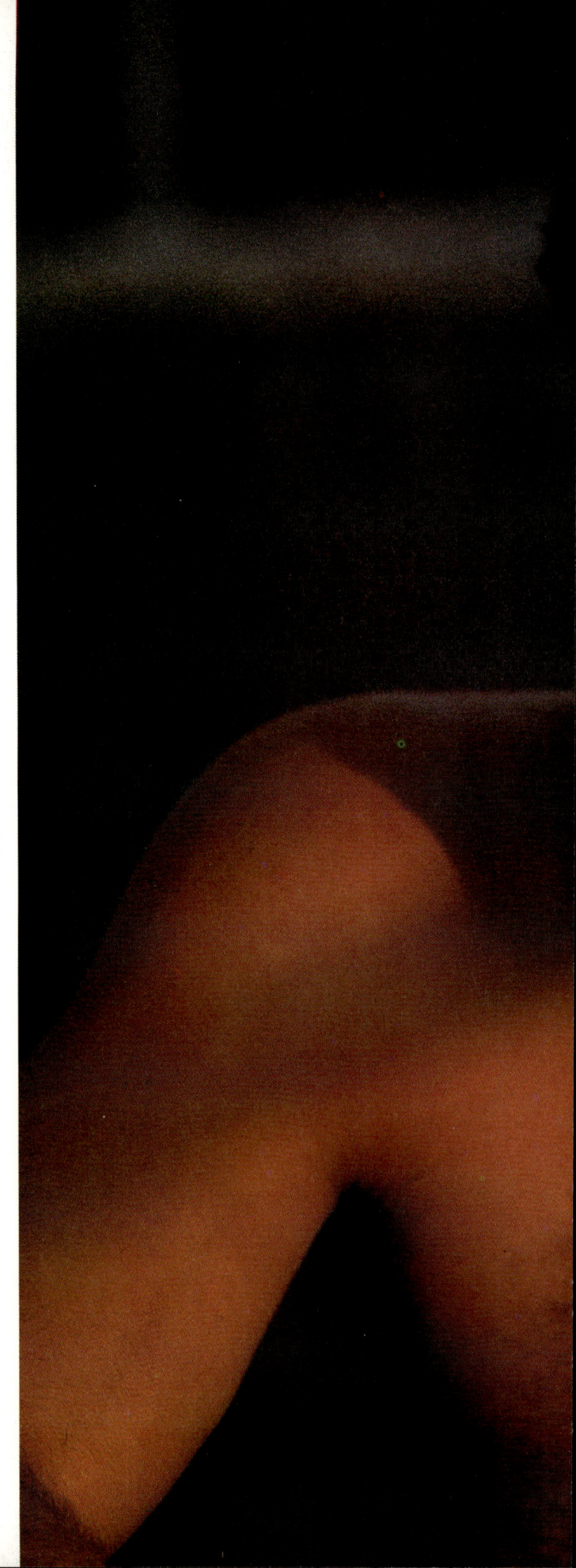

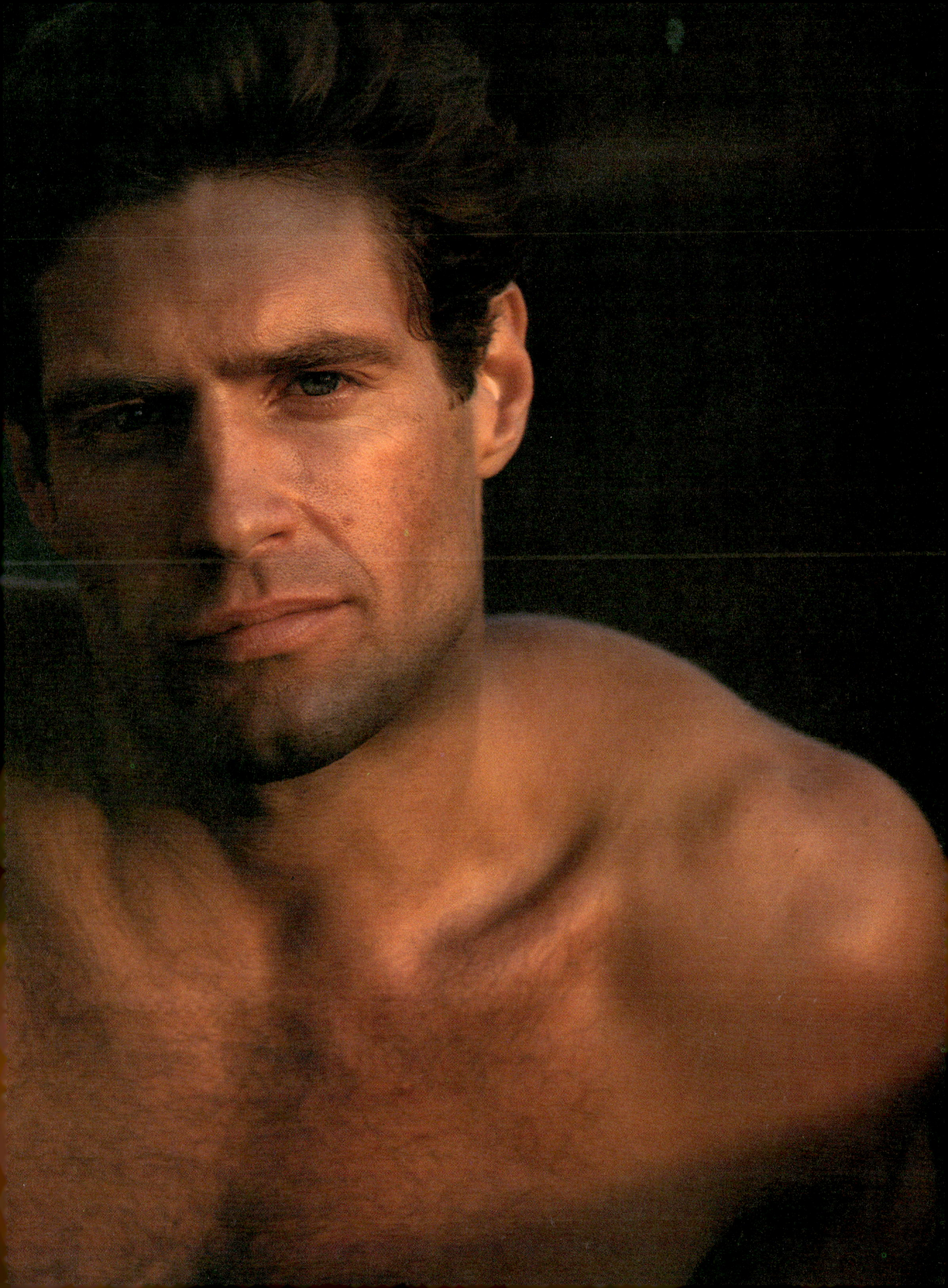

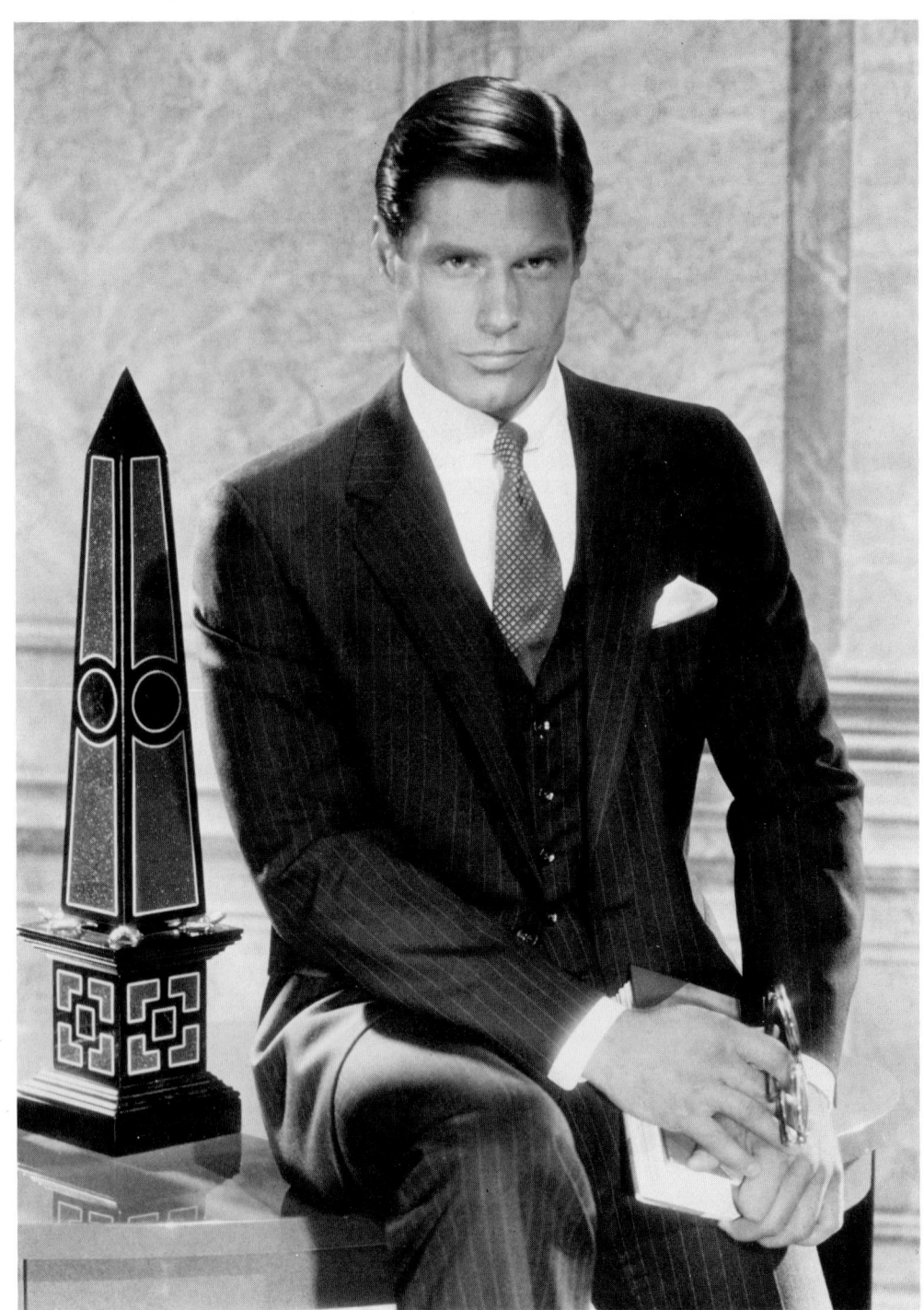

Photograph by Rebecca Blake for Halston

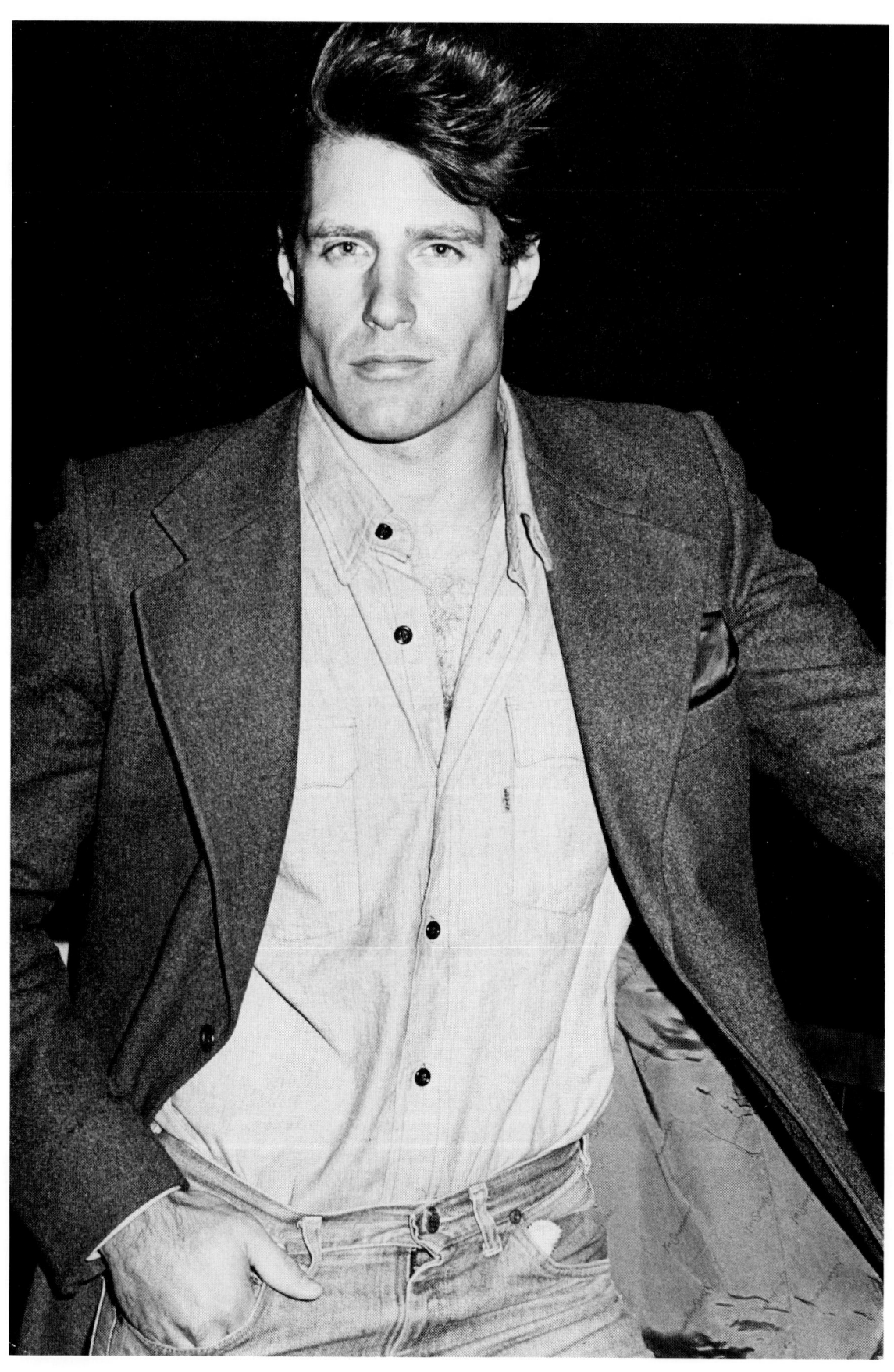

"There's a new breed of men in this industry, and it has nothing to do with sexuality. They are good-looking, intelligent men who have a clear-cut concept of how to do their jobs and make money."

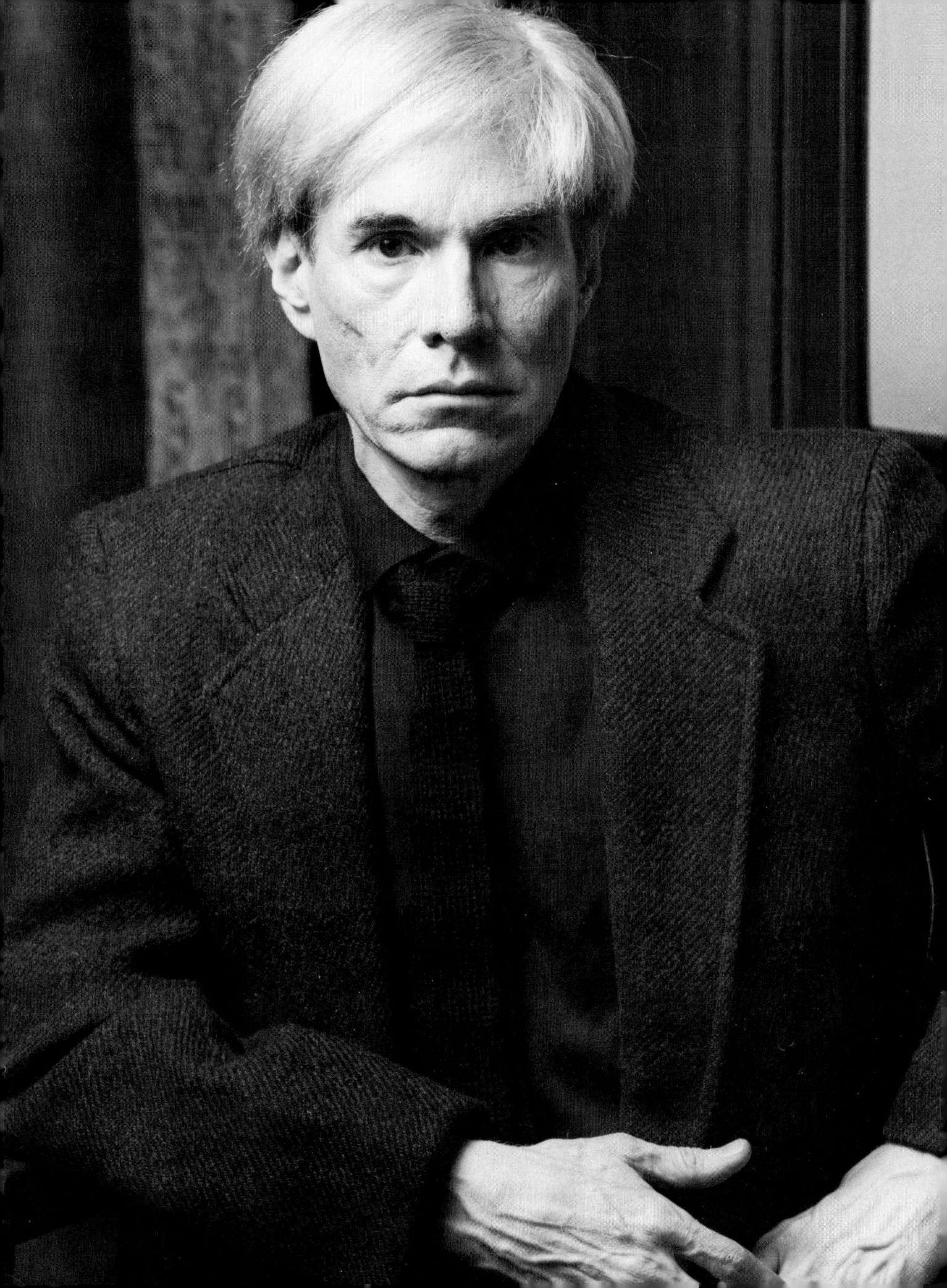

Andy Warhol

As a high-priest of the jet set, Andy Warhol has long traveled in fashion circles. But Andy was usually behind the scenes, capturing popular culture in his art, films, books, and photographs. Since moving in front of the camera in 1982, when he made his debut as a model, Andy has conquered yet another career. Style is no stranger to Warhol, of course. His innovative magazine *Interview,* which he founded in 1974, has often featured new talents and models in exotic photographs. And as his famous Campbell's soup cans demonstrate, Andy has always appreciated the fine art of packaging. Since Andy's distinctive features — snow-white hair and plaintive expression — are uniquely *his,* it was only a matter of time before Andy Warhol, artist and opinion maker extraordinaire, began moonlighting as Andy Warhol, model.

What prompted Andy to enter the competitive world of modeling? "One day," he explains, "the art director of *Interview* asked me if I would like to be represented by Zoli. And I said, 'Yeah, sure, why not?'" Since making that momentous decision, Andy has appeared in a *Vogue* spread and an ad for Barney's, among others, and he has participated in several runway shows. Although it seems as though modeling could not possibly extend Andy's worldwide celebrity, that hasn't been the case. To his delight, his fashion career has made him new fans. "I was in Paris recently and I went to this great men's shop. I was just wandering and this salesman kept staring at me. I assumed he thought I was Andy Warhol or something, but he didn't. He just came up and said, 'Gee, aren't you the model that was in the Barney's ad in *GQ*?' God! That made my day, my week. It made my year."

As he does about every subject, Andy has strong, individual views on fashion, modeling, style, and how they affect American culture. Since Warhol's magazine has elevated the interview to an

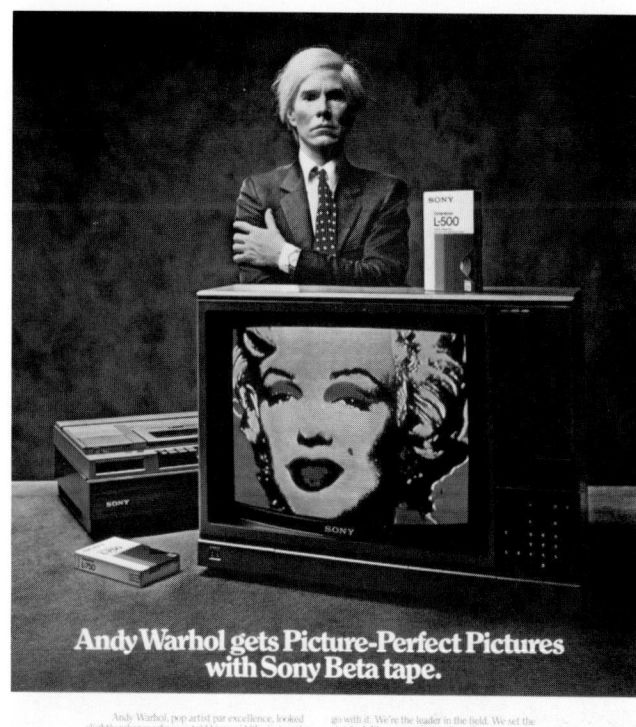

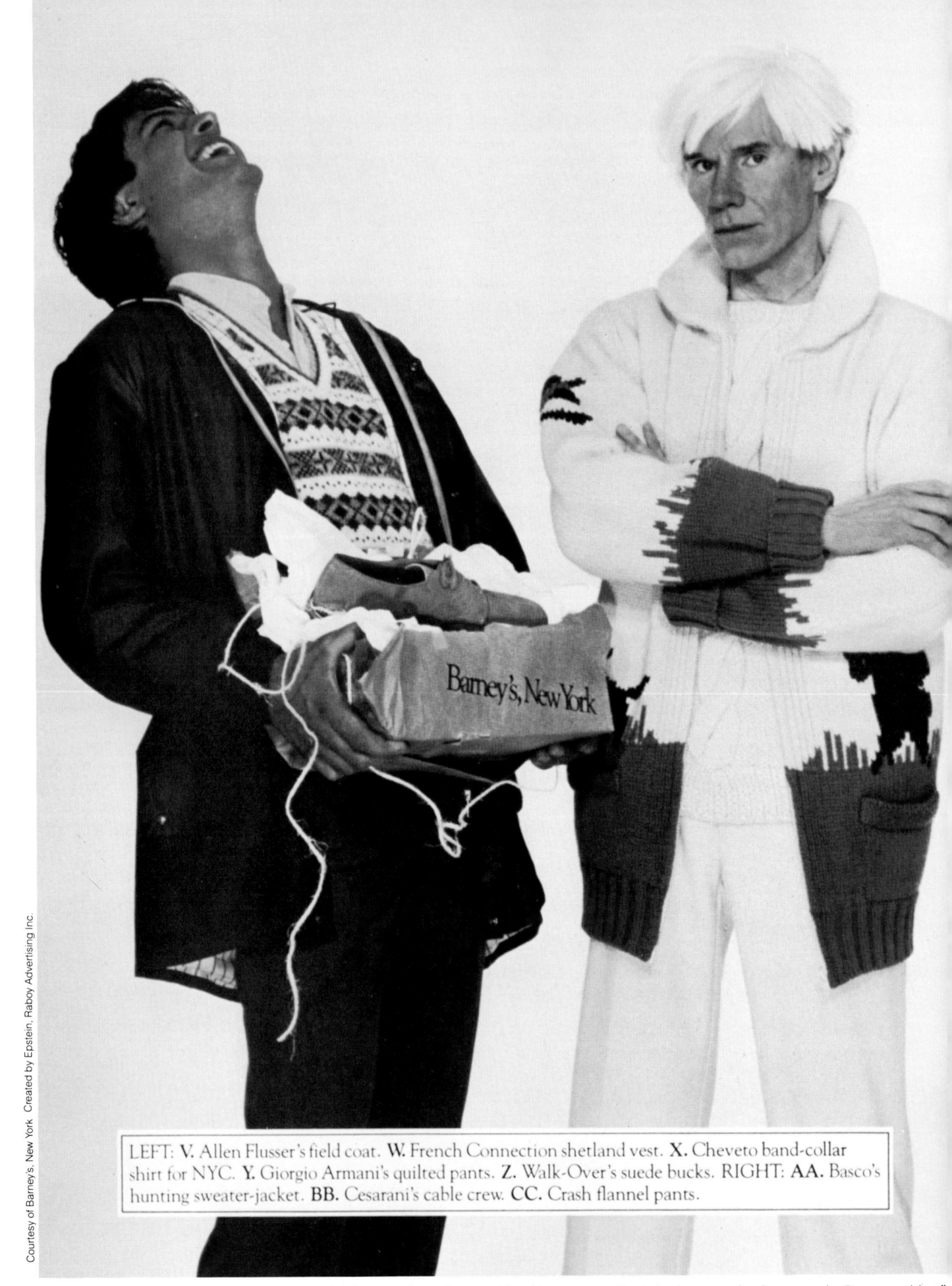

LEFT: **V.** Allen Flusser's field coat. **W.** French Connection shetland vest. **X.** Cheveto band-collar shirt for NYC. **Y.** Giorgio Armani's quilted pants. **Z.** Walk-Over's suede bucks. RIGHT: **AA.** Basco's hunting sweater-jacket. **BB.** Cesarani's cable crew. **CC.** Crash flannel pants.

"I like the sitting around part of being a model. I mean, that's the most fun. You can use the telephone and write a novel. Do something."

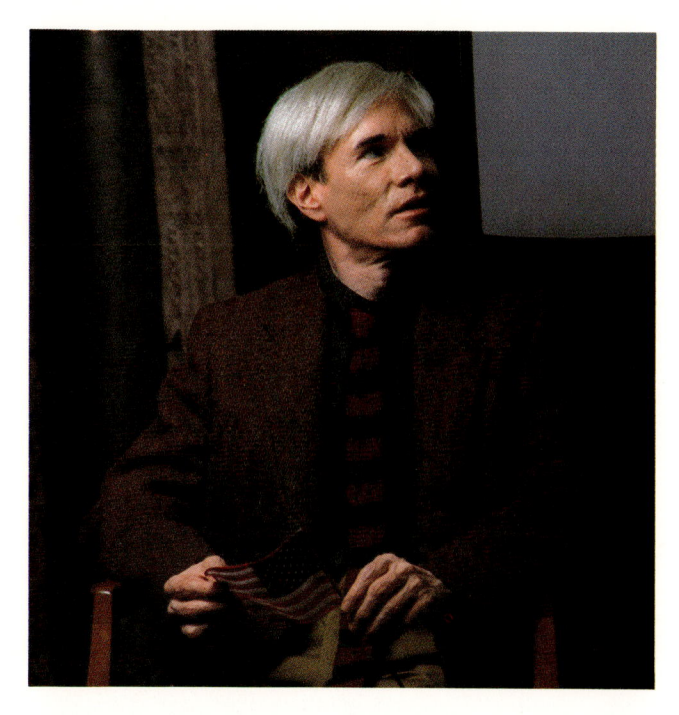

art form, we decided to "model" our talk with Andy after his conversations in *Interview*.

Q: How did you feel in front of the camera the first time?

A: It was sort of easy for *me,* but the poor girl I shot with had to come in at about eight in the morning, and had to have her hair teased for like ten hours. I wish I'd been there that long, because you make more money. They just called me when I had to be there and then shoved me in the picture, and it was over with.

Q: When you go on a job, does someone style you?

A: No, but I want them to. They're all afraid to do anything.

Q: What do you feel that you as a personality do to sell a product?

A: I want to be a comedian. And I decided this is a good steppingstone. Because I just get so nervous, I can't do live TV. I can only do taped TV, and I'm pretty bad at that, but I think I could be a comedian and I thought this is sort of a way to ease into it.

Q: What do you think of the money?

A: It's funny to have these checks dribbling in. I can't wait to do my two-thousand-dollar-a-day job. I want to be in the L. L. Bean or Brooks Brothers catalog.

Q: How do your friends react to your new career?

A: They just don't want to believe it.

Q: Men today, especially young men, are more conscious of the way they look. What do you think of that?

A: Our magazine tried to make that happen. *Interview* tried to make people dress up again. I hate boys with long hair. In this country right now, since there's no war on, everybody's a beauty. It's really scary. They're here because they're not in the Army.

Q: What effect do you think male models are having on the public?

A: Well, everybody's becoming a fashion victim. I mean, if you walk down the street, you see all these trendy kids wearing different jeans. It's amazing that everybody thinks everything is new, but it's all repeat. That's what makes it sort of interesting. I thought drag queens were finished with years ago, and now you go to a party and there's a new drag queen, and it's as if *he* invented it. He doesn't know that drag queens existed before.

Q: Who are your favorite designers?

A: My favorite actually for men is Perry Ellis. I went to his showroom just two days ago. I couldn't believe it. It looks like a billion-dollar showroom. It's so impressive. He had this great coat, and I went to buy it. They said there was only one coat, and it had been sold.

Q: Do you have any Calvin Klein jeans?

A: Well, I have one pair. I collect jeans. I have a Calvin Klein, a Jordache, a Studio 54. I don't wear them. I collect them. The fun thing is to walk down the street and see if you can pick out whose jeans someone is wearing by the design on the back.

Q: How do you dress?

A: I wear the same old things. Levi blue jeans and Lucchese cowboy boots. Brooks Brothers shirts are my favorite. But then I like Paul Stuart clothes, because everything is cotton. Brooks disappoints me a little now: they put polyester in things. I think if you wear the classics, you're safe. They go on forever. But I love the way Halston dresses, because he dresses only in black. Black goes with everything.

Andrew Warhol
Vital & Not So Vital Statistics
Birthdate: "Boys don't have to tell their age anymore."
Height: Medium
Weight: 115 lbs.
Hair: White
Eyes: Blue-gray
Personal Favorites —
Town: Spokane, Washington
Time of Day: 3:41 P.M.
Film: Coming attractions
Actor: Mickey Mouse
Actress: Minnie Mouse
Personal Hero: Walt Disney
Magazine: *GQ*
Hobbies: "Everything I do is a hobby."
Agency: Zoli, New York City

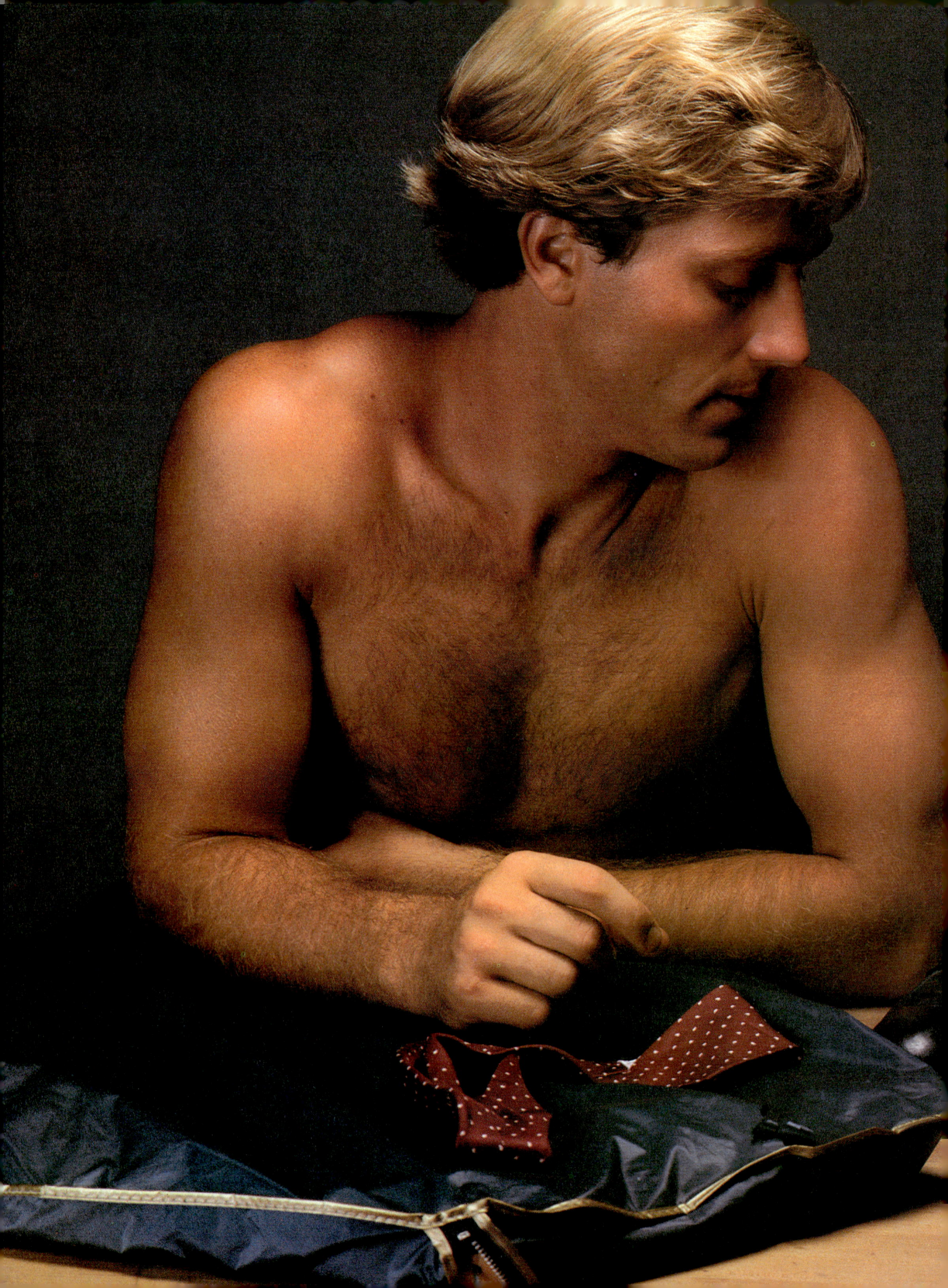

Rich Wiese

Rich Wiese is modeling's resident scholar. While other models quote day-rates, Rich quotes Thoreau and Shakespeare. While others discuss fashion trends, he discusses world politics. "Being a model says so little about what I really am," observes Rich, who is as modest and articulate as he is smart and attractive. "I just don't want to have that stigma, the idea that I'm a pretty face. When I first started, friends at college would see my picture in a magazine, and I'd deny it was me." Even after several seasons in the business, Rich doesn't always admit to his career. If someone asks if he's a model, he may well respond, "Yeah, a model citizen." And, he adds with a laugh, "Even that isn't completely true."

A 1982 graduate of Brown University, Rich majored in geology *and* biology. He was vice-president of Phi Psi fraternity, where his "little brother" was John F. Kennedy, Jr. "On a Saturday morning, our frat resembled a battlefield with bodies strewn all over," Rich reflects. He first experienced the culture shock of entering the fashion world while he was still at Brown. "It was strange," he recalls. "I would fly down from school for a shoot, somebody would pick me up in a limo, and I'd have a hotel room and everything. Then, when it was over, I'd fly back and hitchhike from the airport to my dorm room. That insured that I kept my perspective." And he still has qualms. "Modeling and athletics are probably the only two fields where someone who is completely devoid of any cranial capacity can rise to the very top. It's hard to deal with. I used to commute two hours from my parents' house into New York City, and I'd read the paper on the train. At work, I'd ask if anyone had heard about the NATO decision in Spain. Someone would say, 'No, but did you see who was on the cover of *People*?' I felt sort of alienated."

Rich's rosy-cheeked, robust all-American looks are extremely popular, and the wholesome virtues

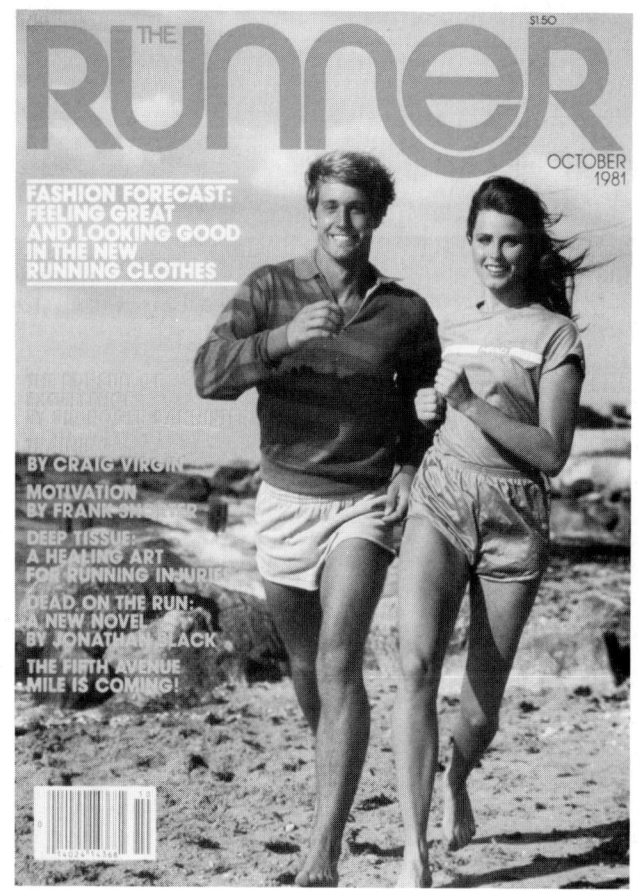

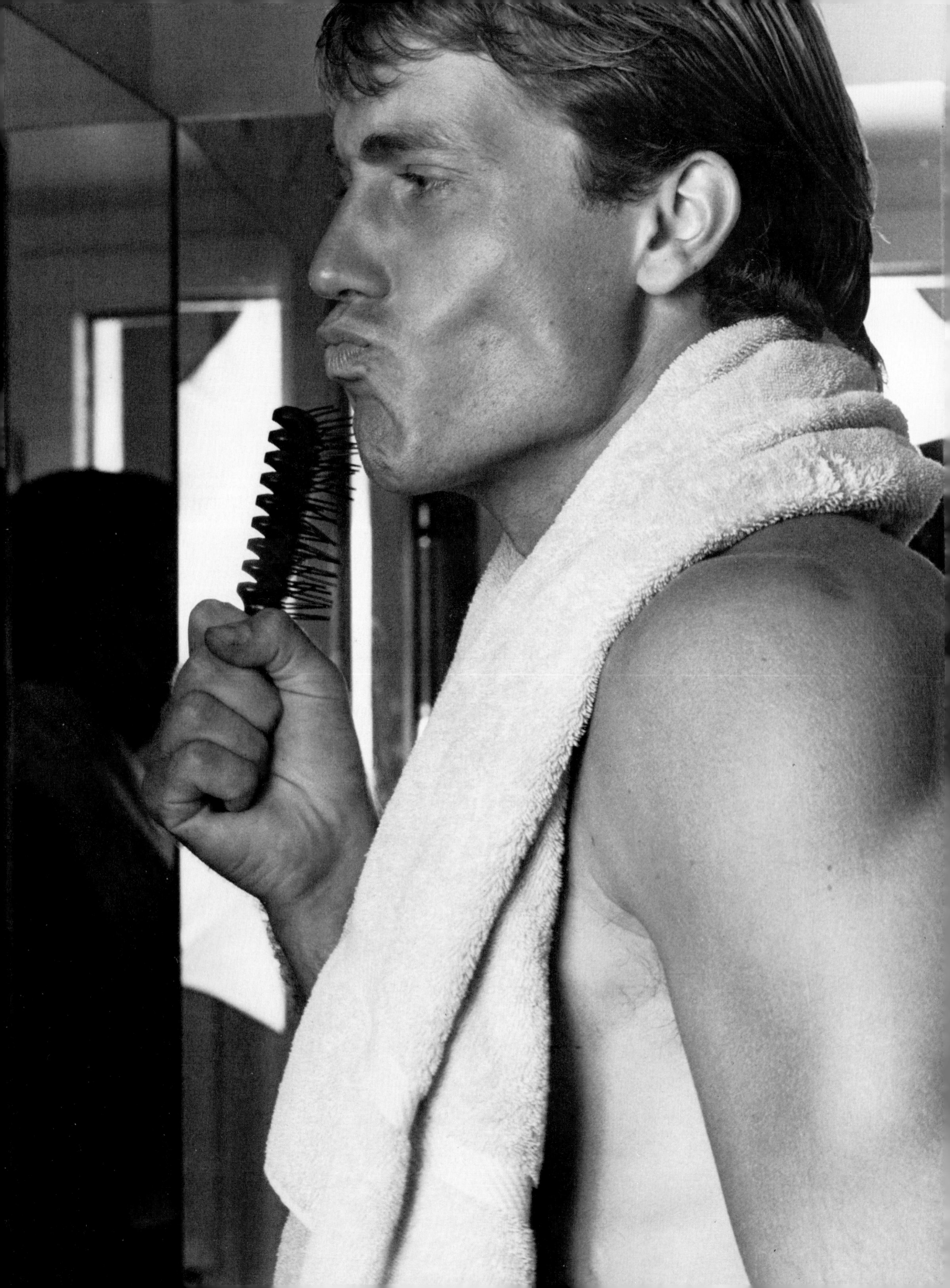

❛
I got a really big kick out of
meeting some of the fashion people when
I first started. Somebody like Cheryl Tiegs.
I'd act very cool and nonchalant about it,
and then when I'd go home to my friends,
I'd say, 'WOW!'
❜

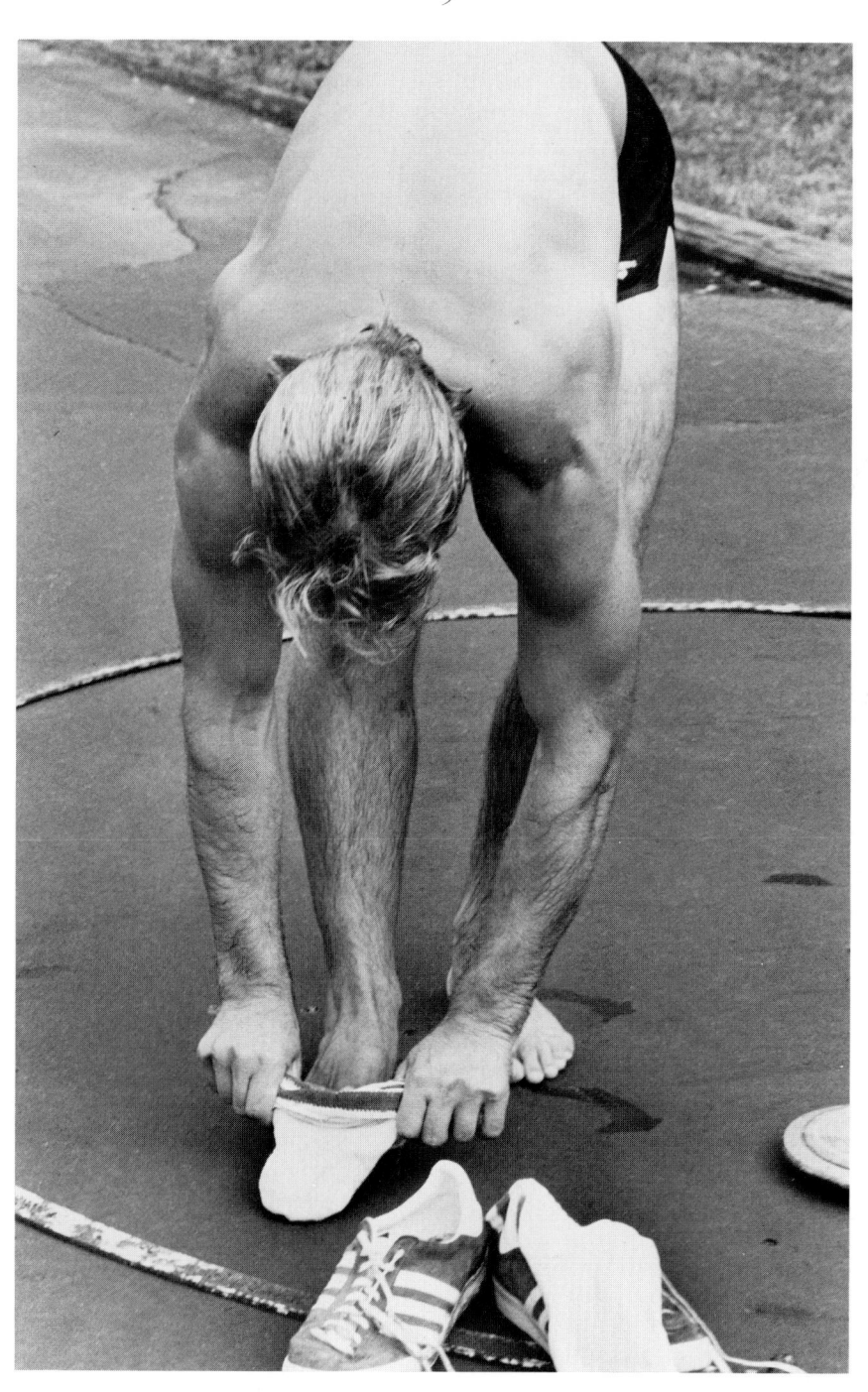

that his face reflects are indeed the values he grew up on. The son of a Pan Am airline captain, Rich was raised in the small town of St. James on Long Island. "I grew up in a traditional Italian family. Every Sunday we would have eighteen or so relatives for dinner. Lots of food and noisy conversation. I enjoyed that. My family is still very important to me." According to Rich, he enjoyed "a very normal childhood. I grew up in a town with less than a thousand people. I went to an all-boys Catholic high school, and I was brought up in an academic environment. I never knew *anyone* in the fashion field. It's not just that I *look* all-American. I *was* an all-American type. I did well in school and sports and had three dogs."

In fact, Rich did so well in high school sports that twice he was named to all-American teams — for javelin throwing and the decathlon. In 1982, he took a gold medal in the Empire State Games handball competition. Rich describes himself as "a jock of all trades," and he even chose his current agency because it had a softball team. Athletics got him into the business. "I was a sophomore at Brown, and I'd just gotten back from a track meet in Bermuda. I walked into the cafeteria with my bags, and I was at the salad bar when a woman walked up to me and asked, 'How would you like to be in *Mademoiselle*?' I said, 'Yeah, right,' and I went to sit down. She came running after me and pleaded, 'Oh, but you'll make so much money.' I asked, 'How much?' At the time, I was a lifeguard making $3.20 an hour. She said, 'Well, how does $125 an hour grab you?'" Now, as a model, Rich finds himself in the curious position of appearing on the covers of sports magazines he read religiously in school.

At some point, Rich intends to trade his modeling career for a journalism career, most likely as a television news anchorman. "Every day is different in that field," he says. "And if you're good at that job, you earn respect. It's very important for me to feel respected." Rich hosted a radio talk show at Brown, where he interviewed Francis Ford Coppola and other celebrities. He also appeared briefly in the movie *Endless Love*. "I just roll around in bed a lot with Brooke Shields." In the best of all possible worlds, Rich would like to be an explorer. He's got a well-thumbed copy of *The Adventurer's Handbook*, and he has climbed Mount Kilimanjaro in Africa as well as dangerous peaks in Alaska, the Alps, and the Himalayas. Rich is also a licensed pilot.

"I've been around. I've had a lot of opportunities," admits Rich. But he has consciously sought variety and he has driven himself hard in search of genuine accomplishment. "There's a quote I always have in the back of my mind," he says. "Thoreau said, 'You're the sum and total of your experiences.' It's my philosophy. Athletics was a chapter in my life, and modeling is another. So many people settle for a mediocre existence instead of going for it."

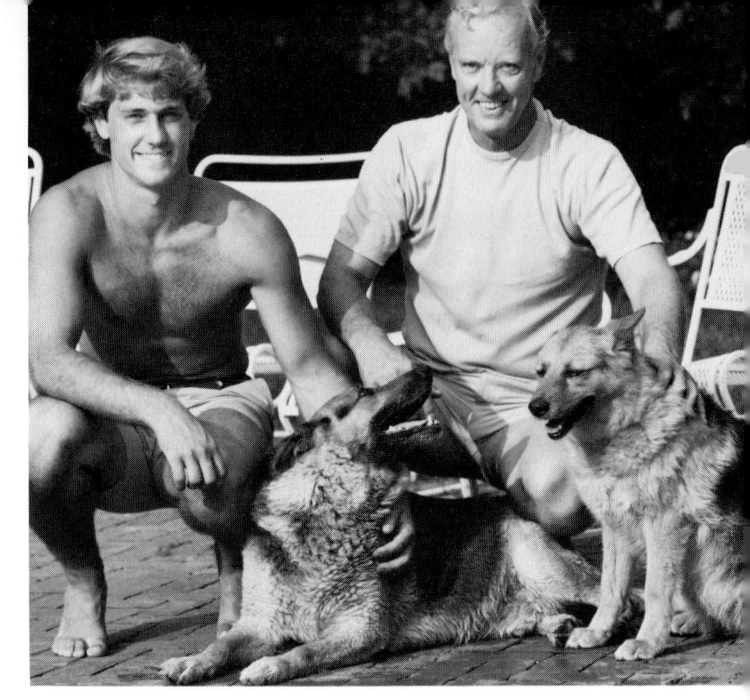

Rich with his father.

Richard C. Wiese
Vital & Not So Vital Statistics
Birthdate: July 13, 1959
Height: 6'1"
Weight: 185 lbs.
Hair: Blond
Eyes: Green
Personal Favorites —
Sport: Baseball
Color: Green
TV Show: *ABC's Nightline,* with Ted Koppel
Snack: Macadamia nuts
Music: Light rock; Rolling Stones; Beach Boys; Simon and Garfunkel; The Police
Sound Track: *The Sound of Music*
Secret Fantasy: "To be a Von Trapp"
Hero: Anwar Sadat
Actor: Robert Redford
Movies: *The Sound of Music; Casablanca; Dr. Zhivago*
Drink: Apple cider, unfiltered
Designer: Ralph Lauren
Dress Style: Baggy shorts and all-cotton T-shirts
Hobbies: Photography; athletics; motorcycles; astronomy; biology; scuba diving
Ideal Woman: Combination of Katharine Hepburn, Ingrid Bergman, and Grace Kelly
Ambition: "To be healthy, wealthy, and wise"
Food: "Unequivocally Italian food" — pasta, scungilli, and tripe
Hangouts: Southampton beach; and Puglia, Jim McMullen's, George Martin, and Joe Hunter's Place, all in New York City
Agency: Ford, New York City

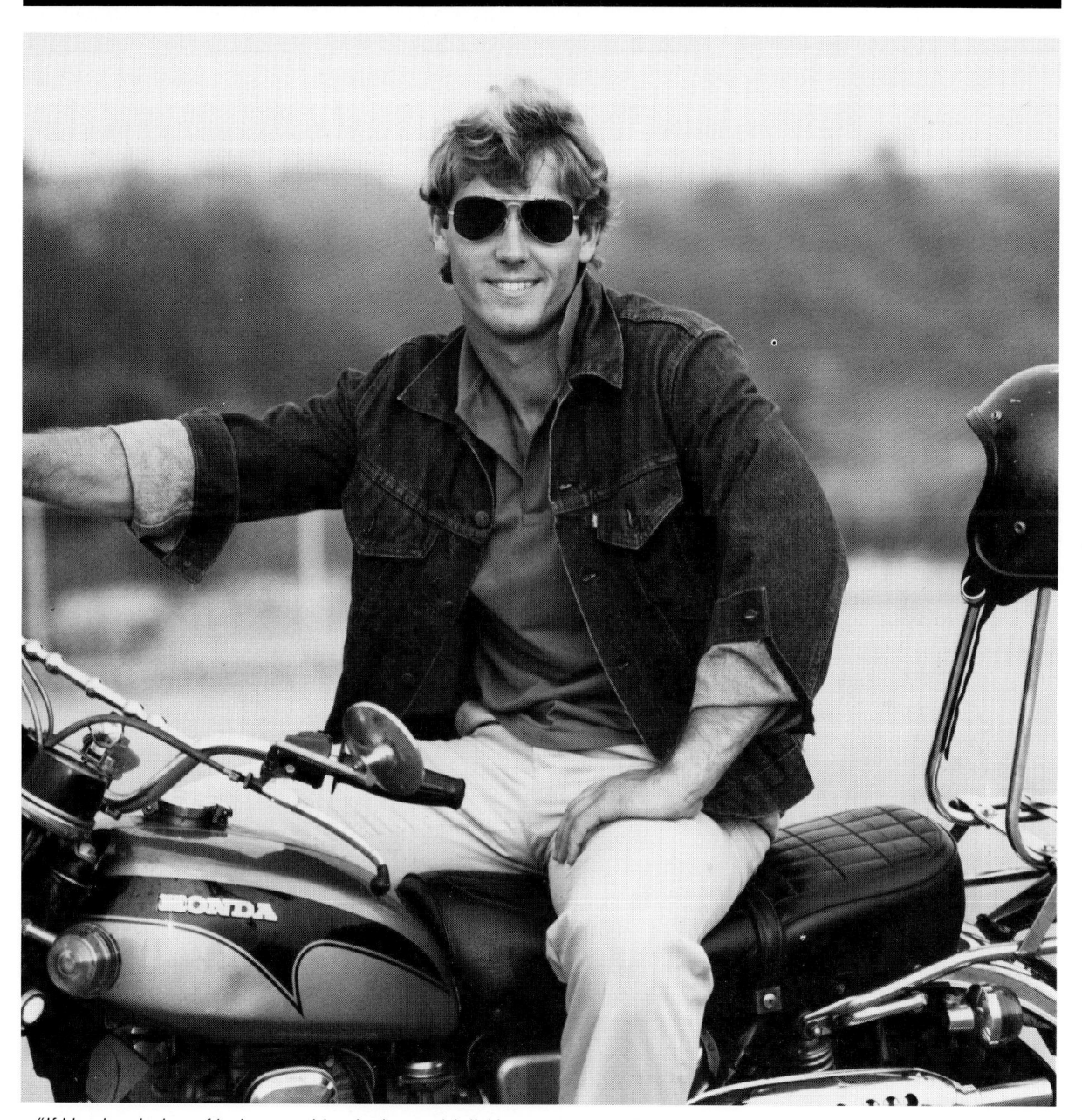

"If I had a choice of being anything in the world, I'd be an explorer. But I guess those days are kind of over."

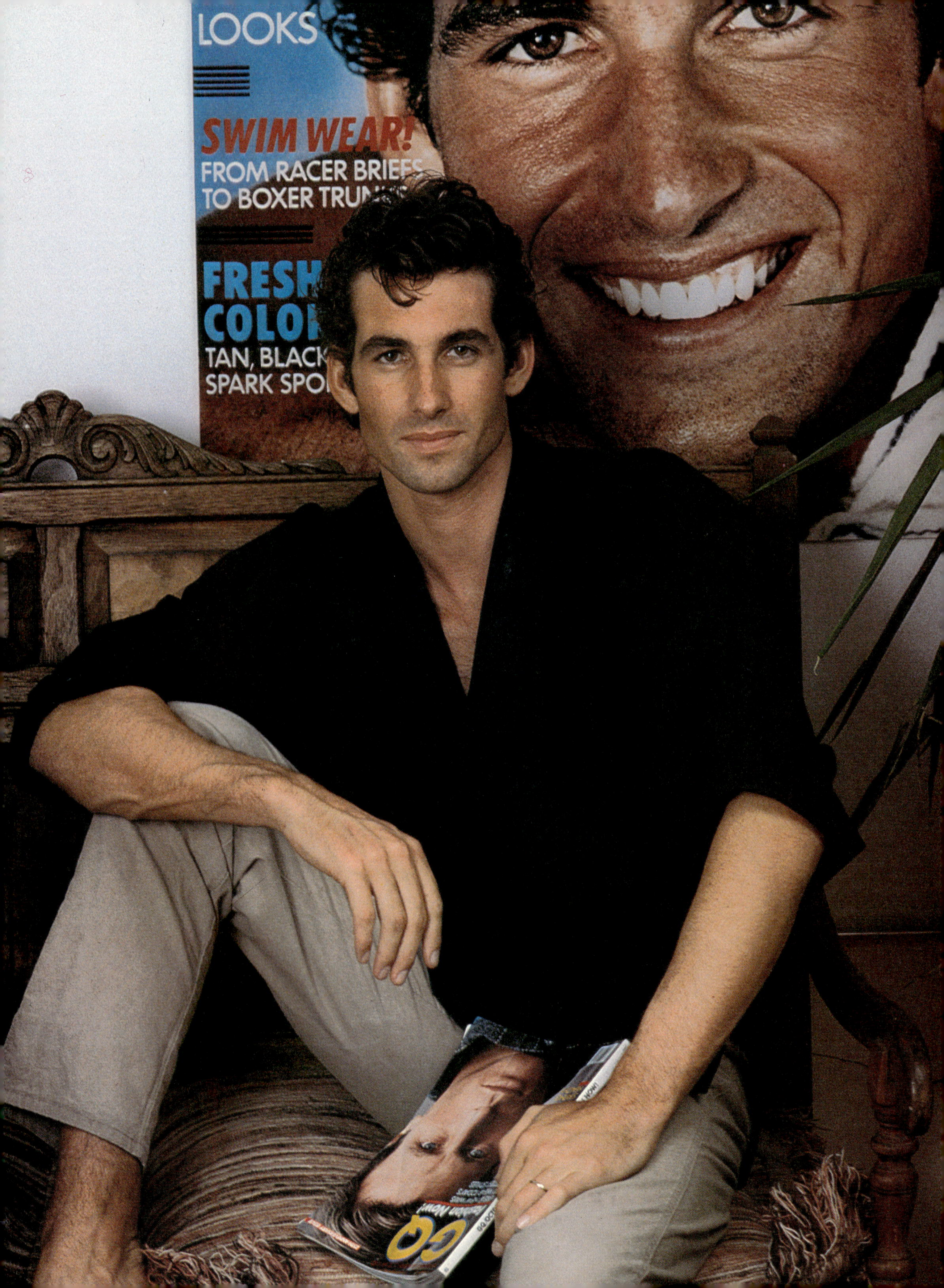
LOOKS
SWIM WEAR!
FROM RACER BRIEF
TO BOXER TRUN
FRESH
COLO
TAN, BLACK
SPARK SPO
GQ

Bill Curry

Billy Curry was the model nobody wanted. When Bill entered the business in 1978, he was routinely rejected by agencies and clients who court him today. But those dismissals didn't deter Bill. "I'd test shoot with anybody who would pick up a camera," he says. "Friends, photographers, hairdressers." And, in retrospect, Bill views those bad days as the foundation of the good days that lay ahead. "People want to see how determined you are. If you stop after the fourth day of rejection, you're never going to get anywhere. The business is full of rejection, every day. That's the name of the game."

Bill was a case of the right guy at the wrong time. When he began modeling, the thirtyish high-fashion type was in demand, and Bill was considered too young for many jobs. Then, suddenly, with the arrival of Jeff Aquilon, the ideal was a beefy, youthful, all-American look, and Bill was considered too old. To propel himself to the top, Bill learned "to become everything to everybody for the moment." He learned the advantages of transcending typecasting. Bill's trademark is no trademark. "You have to be a chameleon in this business," he says. "I've learned to walk the line. It's amazing how you can make yourself look older or younger or just different. You have to learn to adjust yourself rapidly. By feeling the part, you can vary your levels of sophistication."

For a man of many faces, Bill's own background is appropriately diverse, his interests an unlikely combination of down-home and upscale pursuits. Born in York, Pennsylvania, Bill grew up in West Virginia and Ohio. A psychology student at Ohio State University, from which he graduated in 1976, Bill was also a long jumper on the varsity track team. Following college, he worked in a variety of positions: track coach, waiter, landscaper, surveyor, and finally, United Airlines flight attendant.

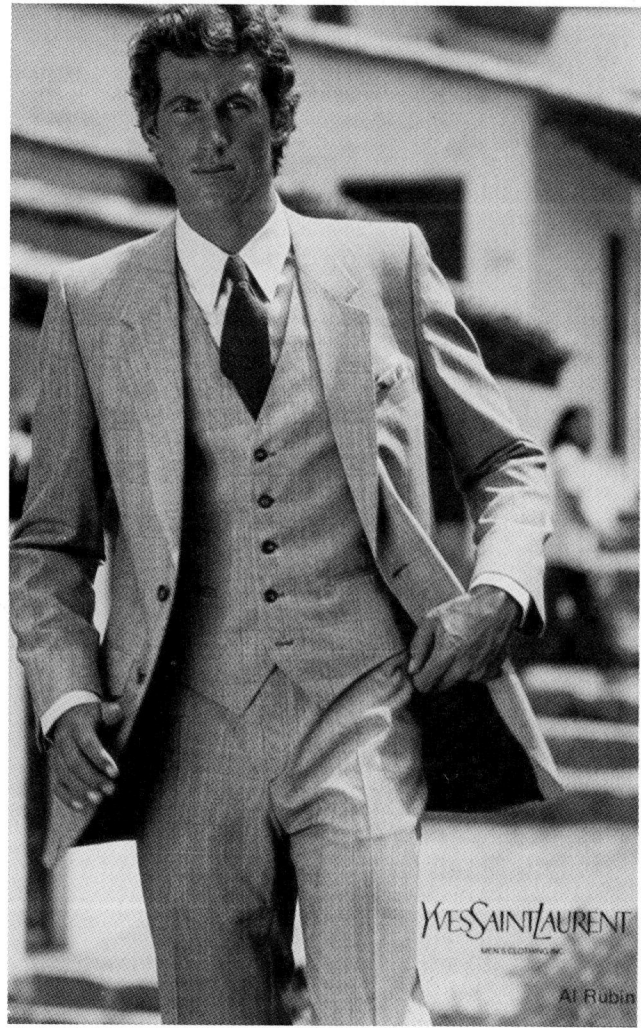

When an ear infection grounded him, Bill turned to modeling.

Although he's often photographed in a suit and a smile, the real constant in Bill's work is a comfortable, at-home-anywhere elegance; he often looks like the city slicker in a country setting. And indeed, Bill's life-style is a mix of city living and outdoor hobbies. Bill lives in New York's Greenwich Village, but as frequently as possible, he indulges "my first two loves: the ocean and fishing." At least three times a year, he travels to Montana for trout fishing. "There's no other job in the world that would let me do that," he says. And if he's not trout fishing in the West, he may be scuba diving in the Caribbean. "I started diving about three years ago. I've always loved the ocean, and I wanted to be a marine biologist as a kid. But since we lived inland, I had to give that up. Scuba diving has introduced me to a whole new world." In fact, Bill wants to continue his exploration of that world by making underwater documentaries with his diving colleagues. "We want to make people aware of the plight of the ocean," he says.

Bill's cultured side is evident in his burgeoning art collection, which evolved out of a modeling trip to Europe. Indeed, such a trip was one of his prime motivations for choosing this career. "I'd always wanted to work my way across Europe as a model," he says. "I went to Greece, Milan, then to Florence and Rome and Venice and Sardinia. Switzerland, Zurich, and Hamburg, Germany. I planned each city and stayed a month, modeling to pay for my food and hotels. Going to Europe was the greatest experience of my life. I was exposed to great wealth and to great poverty, and I learned an incredible amount." Bill was especially impressed with the legendary art of Florence and Paris, and he began both a study of art history and a private collection, which now includes German sculpture, primitive African art, Haitian pieces, and Jamaican art. There's a musical side to Bill as well: his brother Jack is an expert musician and Bill's plan is to produce his brother's records in the near future.

Despite the initial obstacles and resistance he encountered, Bill maintains great appreciation for his career. Among other things, it has helped him develop his own peculiar fashion sense, which is marked by a penchant for the layered look. "I don't dress like my pictures," says Bill. "I like crazy combinations. What I like to do is take six pieces of clothing that look like they could never go together and make them look great." Bill also enjoys the camaraderie of the business. "It's a great feeling when I'm in a foreign city and don't know anyone and pick up a magazine and see Rick Edwards or somebody in it. I just laugh and think how I know

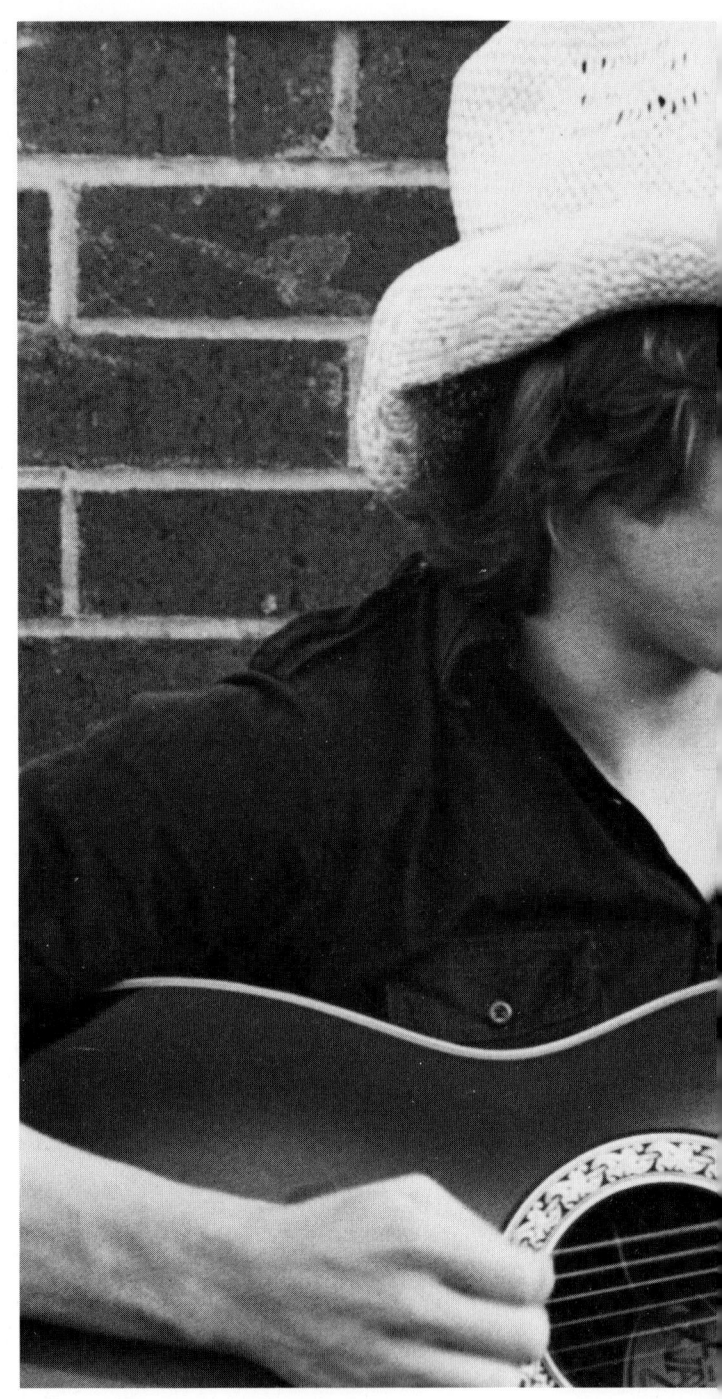

Bill jamming with his brother Jack.

these guys as they *really* are. It's like being back on the track team in college." What modeling has primarily taught Bill is the rewards of patience and perseverance. "There's more to modeling than good pictures and looking good," he says, relaying the advice he often gives aspiring models. "It has to do with sticking it out and believing in yourself. For some kids, modeling can be a real trap and you end up with only a boxful of pictures. You have to learn one basic thing: use this business and don't let it use you."

❛

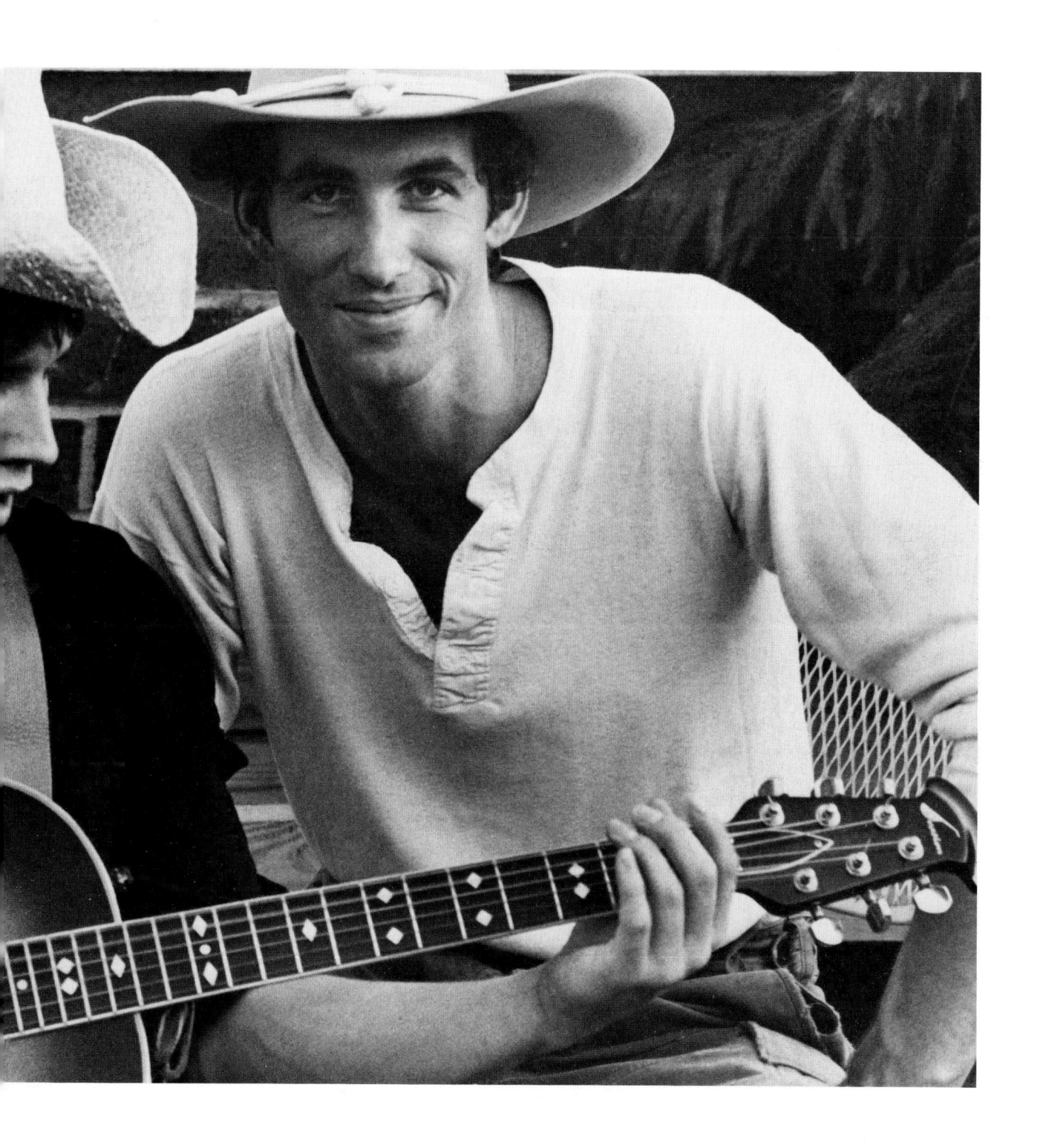

For years,
I wanted a GQ *cover*, a real tough look, with a five-days' growth,
like a mountain man. Then, when I finally got a cover,
it was me smiling.
Now everybody wants me smiling.
I'm so tired of smiling.

❜

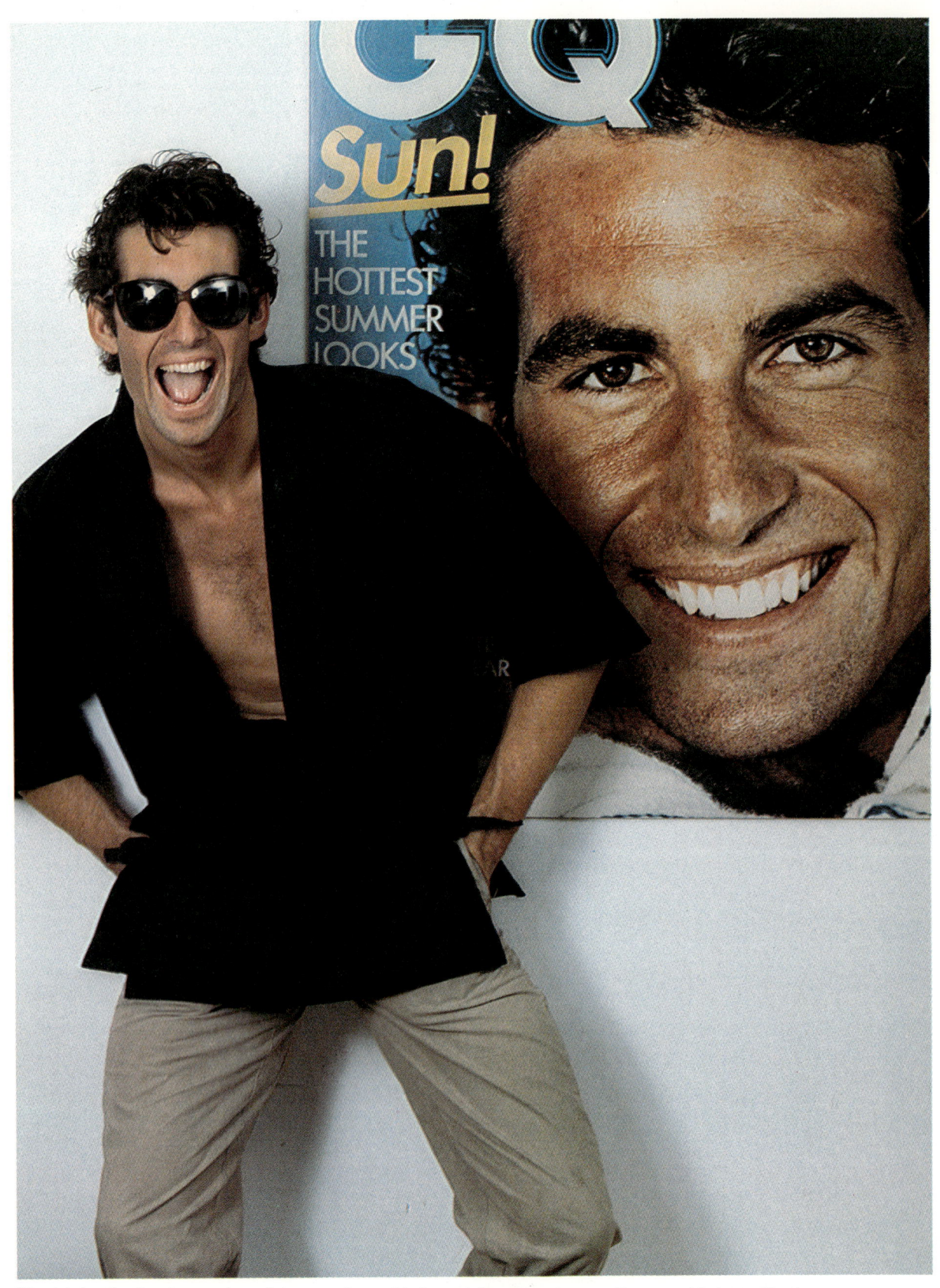

"Sophistication is a learned art. I'm not really sophisticated. I'm a regular guy. For a sophisticated look, the photographer only has to freeze that image and attitude for one frame."

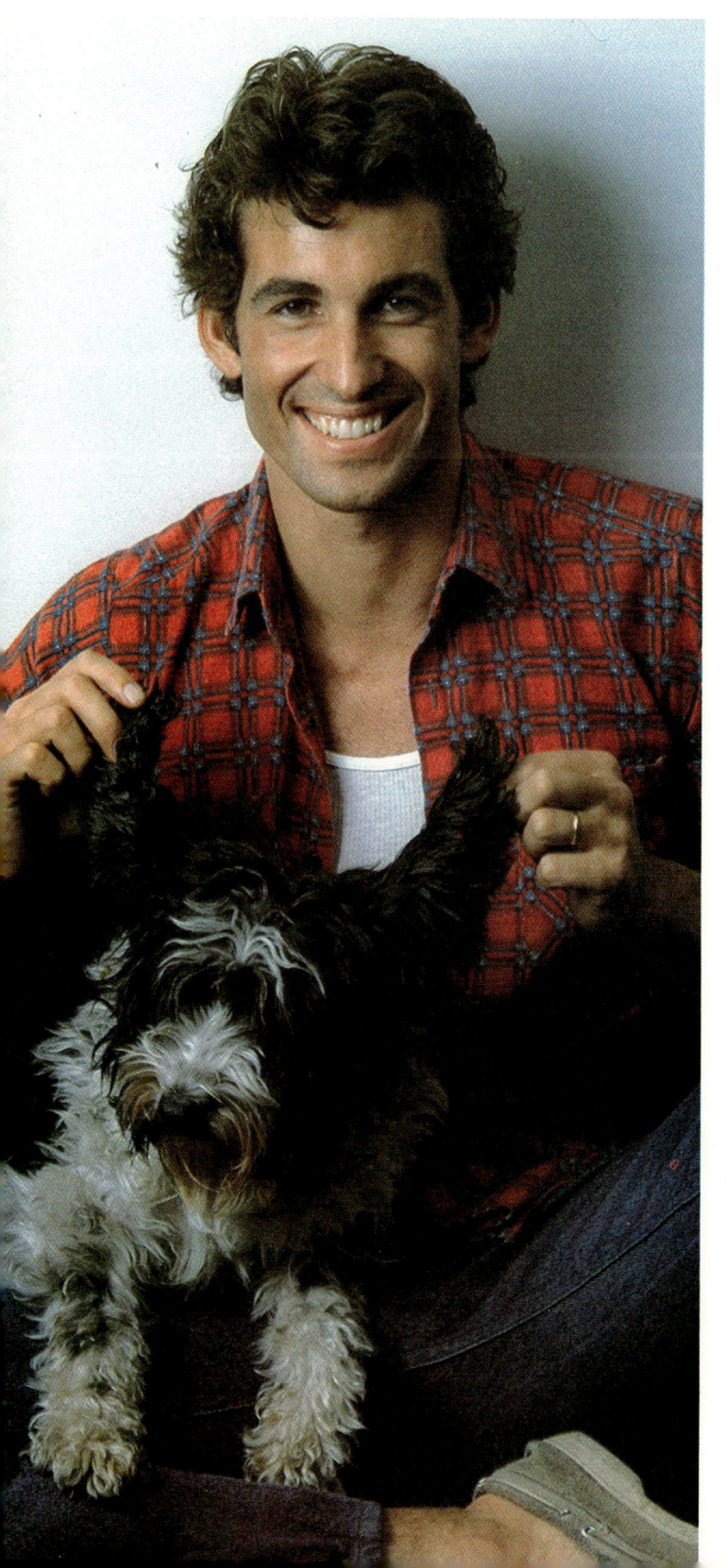

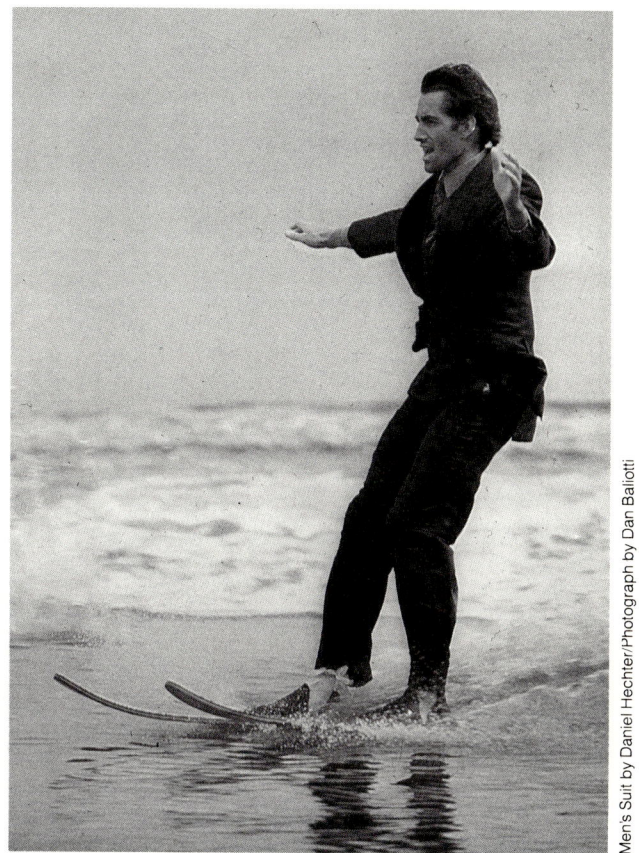

Men's Suit by Daniel Hechter/Photograph by Dan Baliotti

Bill Curry
Vital & Not So Vital Statistics
Birthdate: January 8, 1954
Height: 6'1"
Weight: 170 lbs.
Hair: Brown
Eyes: Brown

Personal Favorites —
Town: Port Antonio, Jamaica
Time of Day: Evening at sunset
Color: Blue
Snacks: Canada Dry ginger ale; smoked almonds
Actors: Clint Eastwood; Sean Connery
Actresses: Ann Archer; Laura Antonelli
Movies: *Little Big Man*; *Swept Away*
Designers: Perry Ellis (U.S.A.); Gianni Versace (Europe)
Magazines: *National Geographic*; *GEO*
Ambitions: "To dive with the whales in Argentina and produce underwater documentaries"
Music: The Spinners; Bob Marley; Dillinger
Dress Style: Army/Navy surplus style, "clothes that are worn and comfortable"
Hobbies: Scuba diving; horseback riding; fishing
Hangouts: Caffe Reggio, The Bagel, Heartbreak Club, all in New York City
Agency: Wilhelmina, New York City

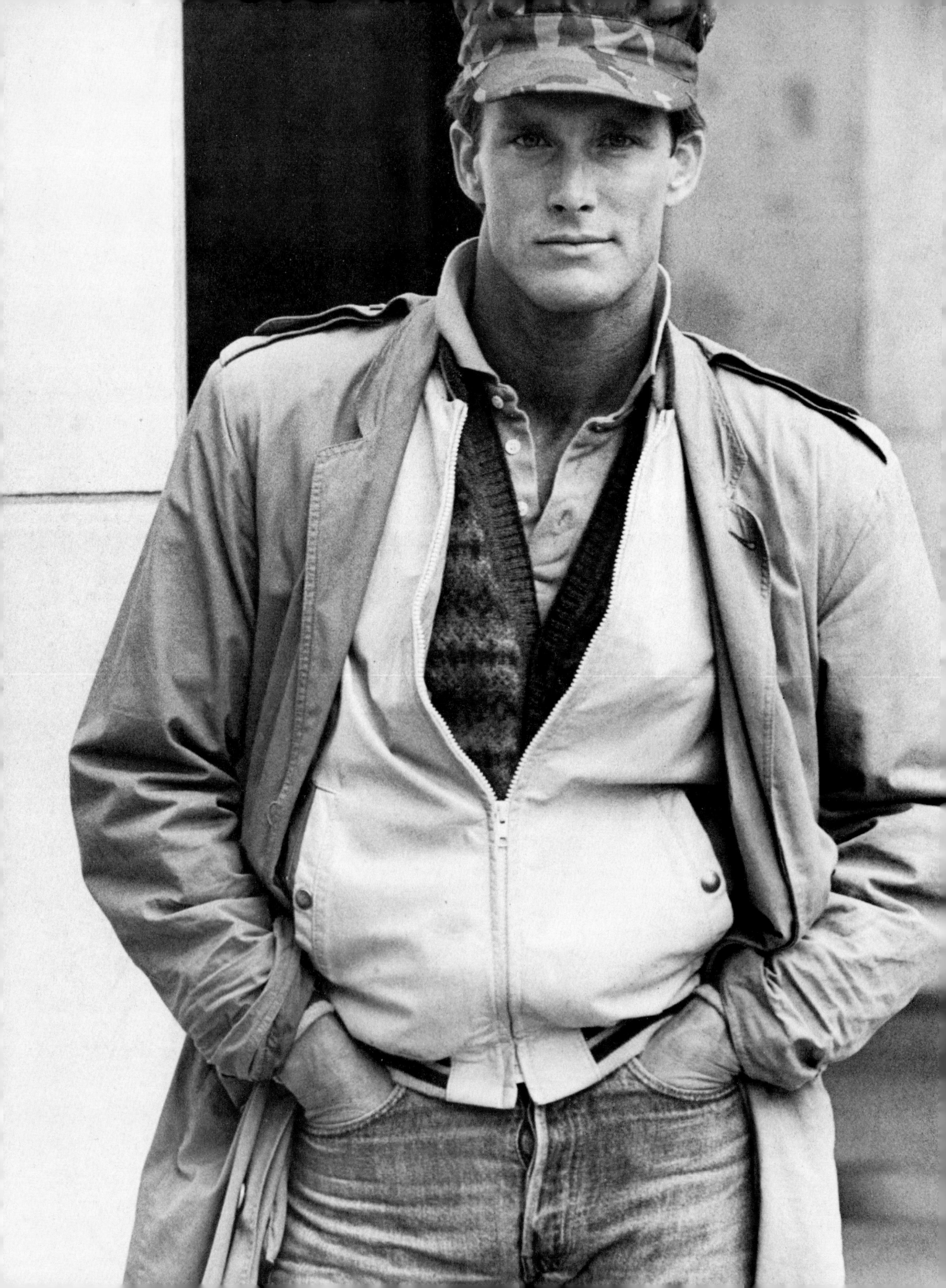

Michael Holder

Michael Holder is both a product and an emblem of his times: the tumultuous 1970s. With high cheekbones and a good build, Michael is a smashing romantic figure, a Heathcliff in blue jeans. Michael's chiseled features epitomize a male ideal that dominated fashion modeling through the 1970s. But, in the early 1980s, Calvin Klein, Bruce Weber, and others revolutionized the industry by introducing athletic men whose looks and demeanors were younger, more all-American, more guy-off-the-street and boy-next-door. The severely elegant type became an endangered species. But with a look that can appear either manly or boyish, suave or impish, Michael has a versatility that transcends any trend. His handsomeness is always fashionable.

Beneath Michael's attractive veneer, there is an articulate, intelligent adult who has always been a bit at odds with the polished image he projects. A man who came of age during the Vietnam era, Michael has experienced great ambivalence about his profession, his life-style, and himself. As his sensitive conversation makes clear, the 1970s were an explosive, critical period that shaped Michael's perspective. Says Michael, "I saw the world was not going to be the way my parents had thought, the American dream idea. According to them, you just do everything you're supposed to do and it comes out right in the end. I opted for something different." Because his father was an officer in the Air Force, Michael, who was born in Atlanta, lived in many different places as a child: Japan, France, Germany, Wyoming, and Florida. Finally, the family settled in Louisiana, where Michael spent eight years and graduated from high school. Michael's father was a strict disciplinarian, and the son rebelled at an early age. As he recalls, "I valued anything that my father opposed. I always feel he was disappointed that I didn't become a Baptist minister or a colonel."

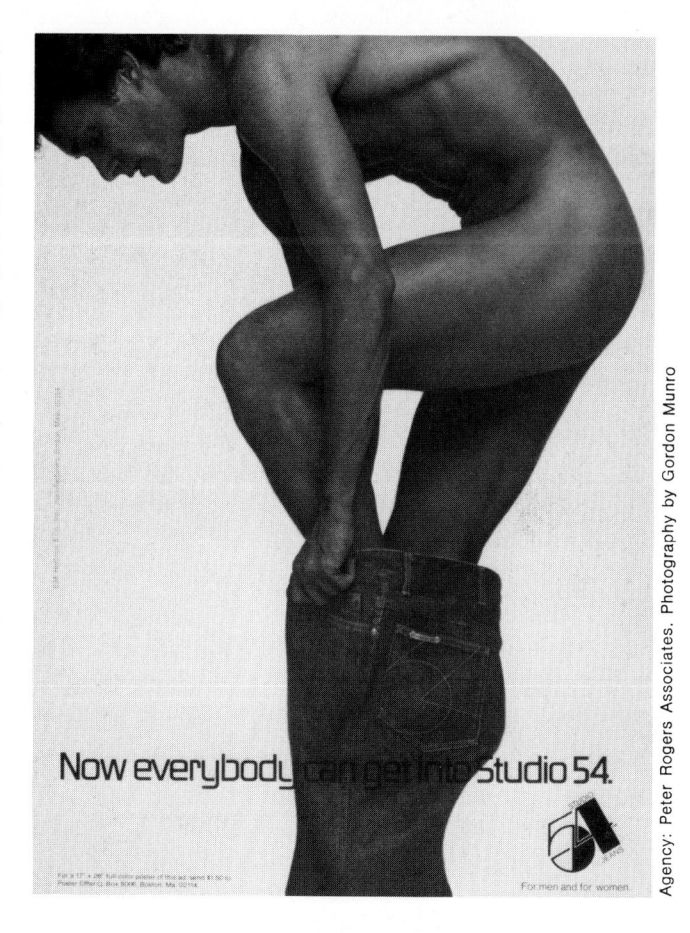

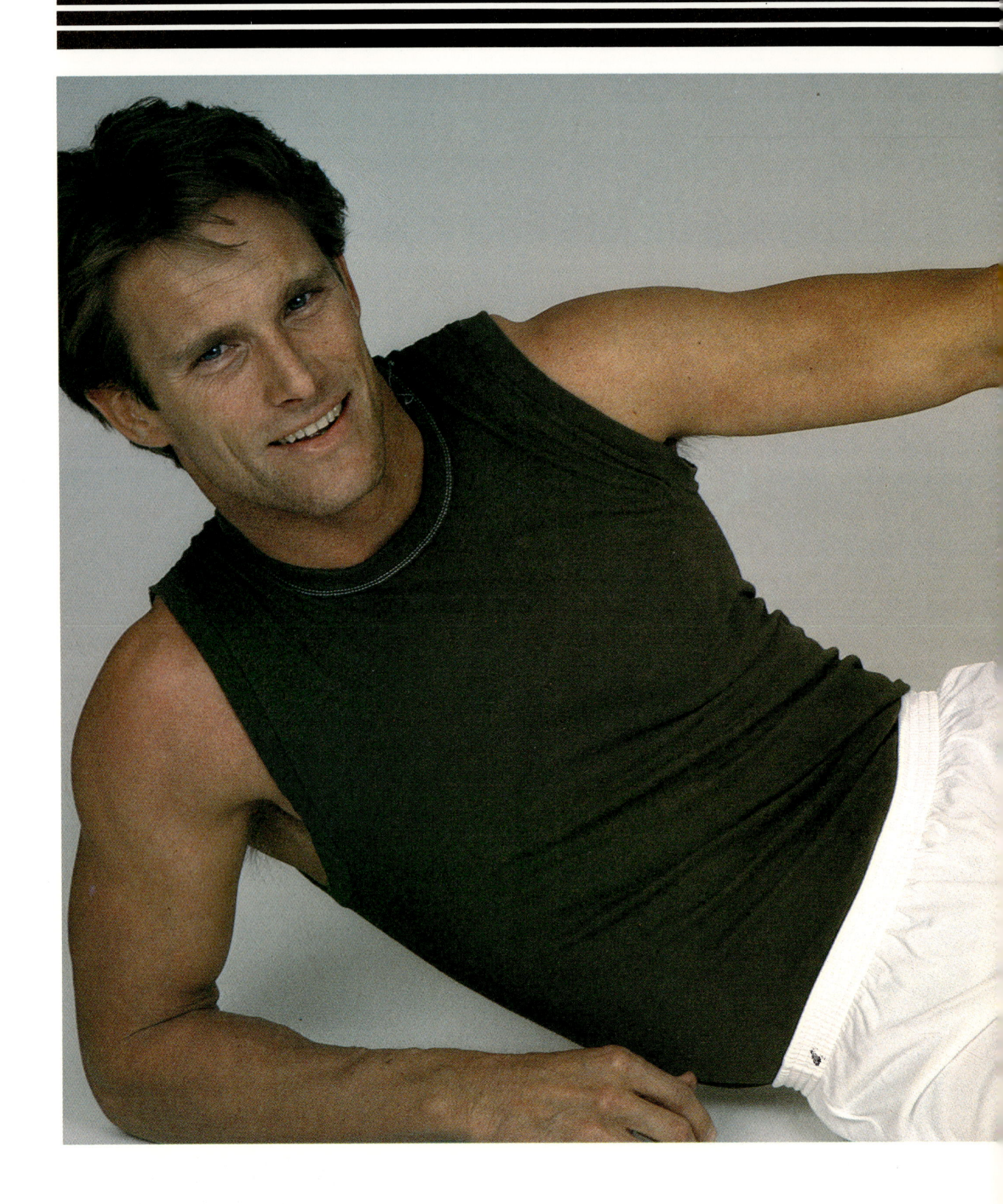

'My first magazine job was an exotic environment with three women considered top models. I thought I was in little-boy heaven.'

Michael still has a predilection for doing the unconventional and saying the unexpected. Despite his enormous success as an industry superstar, he isn't fazed by his wealth. "Money doesn't really change one's life," he says. "It doesn't change the way you think about yourself." And Michael seems remarkably unaware of and unaffected by his handsomeness. "I am totally insecure," he admits. "Usually, I feel like I wish I had a suntan. I wish I were in better shape. I wish I hadn't stayed up so late last night. I wish I were happier and able to project a lot more confidence." Michael considers his good looks — and he attributes his modeling success to his mother's cheekbones — something of a mixed blessing. "I don't think good looks necessarily affect how ambitious you are or how successful you're going to be. It's a burden if you're considered by society to possess good looks, because people feel you haven't had to struggle to prove other things."

Michael has developed his cosmopolitan view of the world through a host of distinctive experiences. His biography is a coast-to-coast litany of odd jobs and good fortune. Because he didn't begin modeling until he was thirty years old, Michael has indeed earned the world-wise look he often assumes in photographs. After graduating from Claremont College with a degree in English in 1969, Michael was commissioned as a second lieutenant in the Army at age twenty-two. The Vietnam War was on, and Michael was in the Medical Service Corps stateside. For two years, he worked in various clinics in Texas and Virginia treating problem cases. Then he left the Army, moved to San Francisco, and worked as a carpenter and a shipyard laborer. He was studying art when a model in his figure class encouraged him to try fashion modeling. He signed with an agency

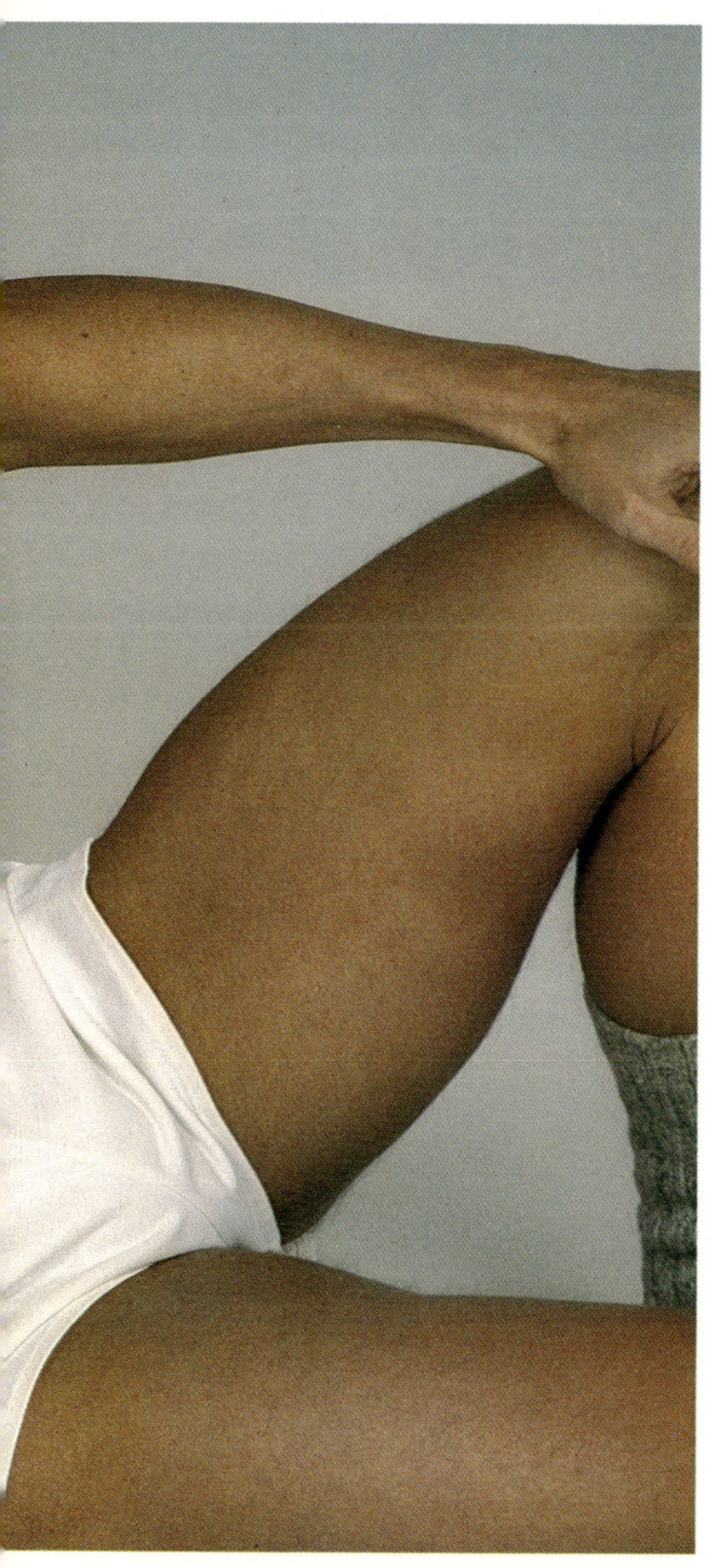

"I've always been very clothes-conscious. Even as a little, kid, I wanted this, I wanted that, and if I didn't get it, I was heartbroken."

Courtesy of Saks Fifth Avenue

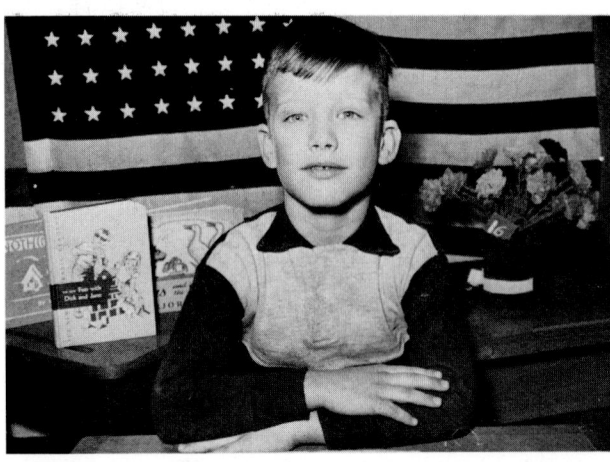

Michael in second grade.

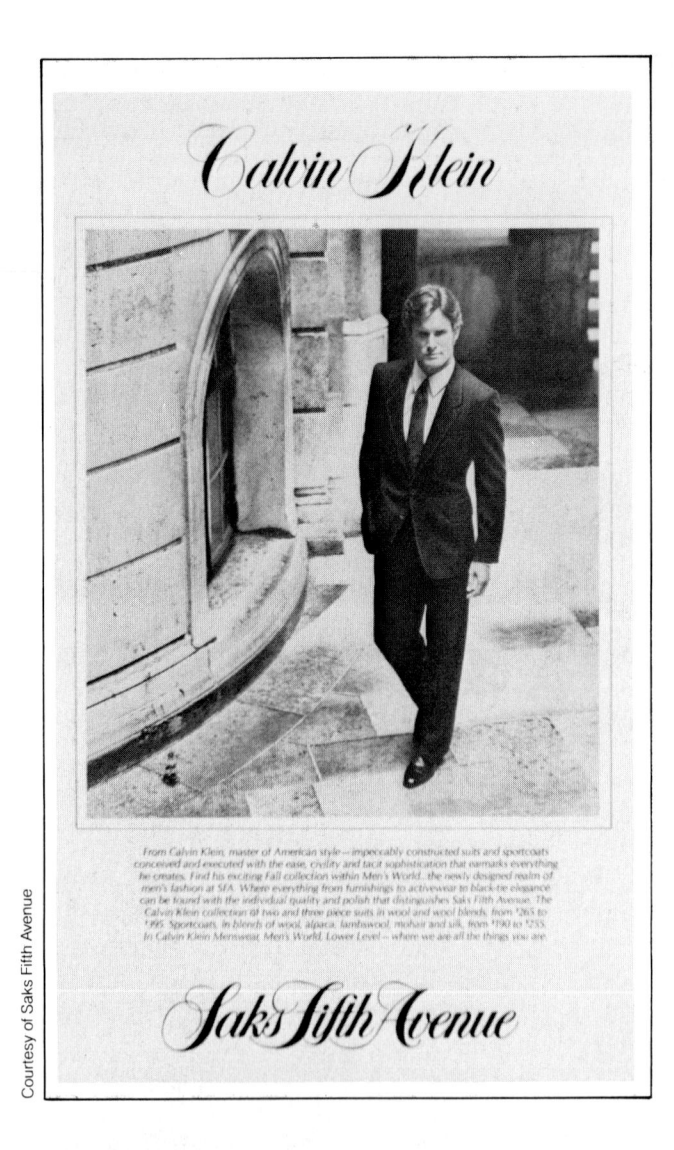

in California, and after success on the West Coast, moved to New York, where his second job was a *GQ* cover. "I was fortunate enough to have good exposure quickly," says Michael. "I never had to go through a period of struggling to make myself believe that there was a career in this. When I started, I think modeling had just begun to become something that was okay for a man to do."

During his occasional free moments, Michael concentrates on his two other interests: acting and keeping in shape. "I average about ten hours a week at the gym," says Michael. "I do a lot of exercises that are particular to me to keep my body balanced. But every day I work on my stomach, and I alternate days working on my legs and back." Michael works just as intently on his acting. He has been studying for several years, and he sees it as the next logical step. "I think acting is an art form that has value. It contributes to a social good. I think I may have a talent for acting, more than I have a talent for modeling."

Despite his ambivalence about his career and his looks, Michael certainly doesn't underestimate the privileges of modeling. "One of the opportunities that modeling offers is that if you want to do something, you can find the time. It allows you room. I make time for things that are important to me, like reading, sketching, talking to friends or a shrink. I also keep myself healthy, whether it's taking a vacation to get some sun or working out at the gym. If you have a lot of things to do, you seem to be able to fit more in. You get energy from using yourself."

Michael Holder

Vital & Not So Vital Statistics
Birthdate: June 9, 1947
Height: 6′
Weight: 165 lbs.
Hair: Light brown
Eyes: Blue

Personal Favorites —
Book: *Brave New World*
Town: New York City
TV Show: *The Little Rascals*
Comic: *Sad Sack*
Hero: Ham, first U.S. chimpanzee-astronaut
Magazine: *Vogue*
Athlete: Mikhail Baryshnikov
Actor: James Woods
Actress: Susan Sarandon
Cereal: Sugar Pops
Drink: Fresh squeezed grapefruit juice with vodka
Time of Day: Any time of day when you can see a crescent of the moon in the sky
Hobbies: Sex; rock and roll
Agency: Zoli, New York City

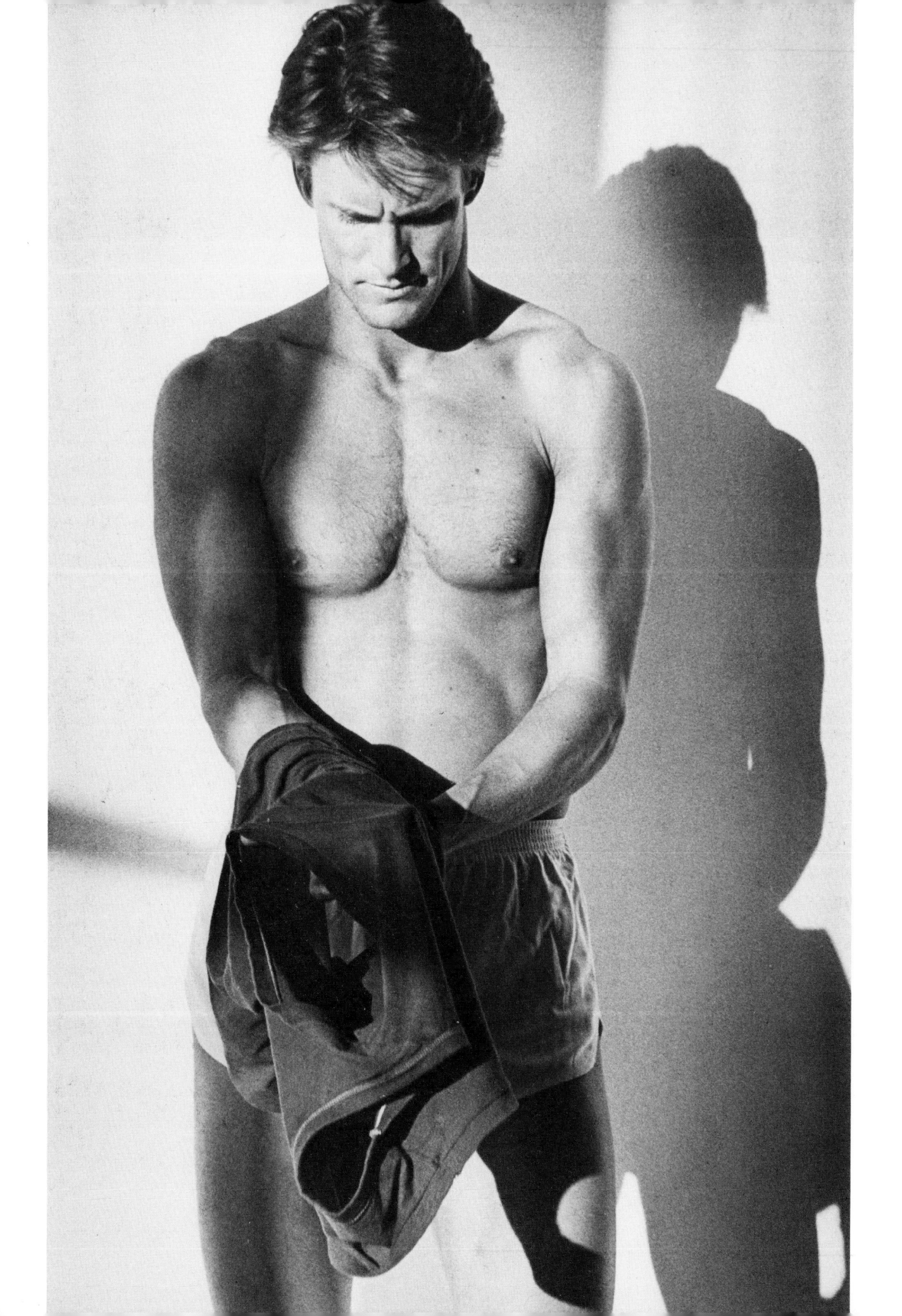

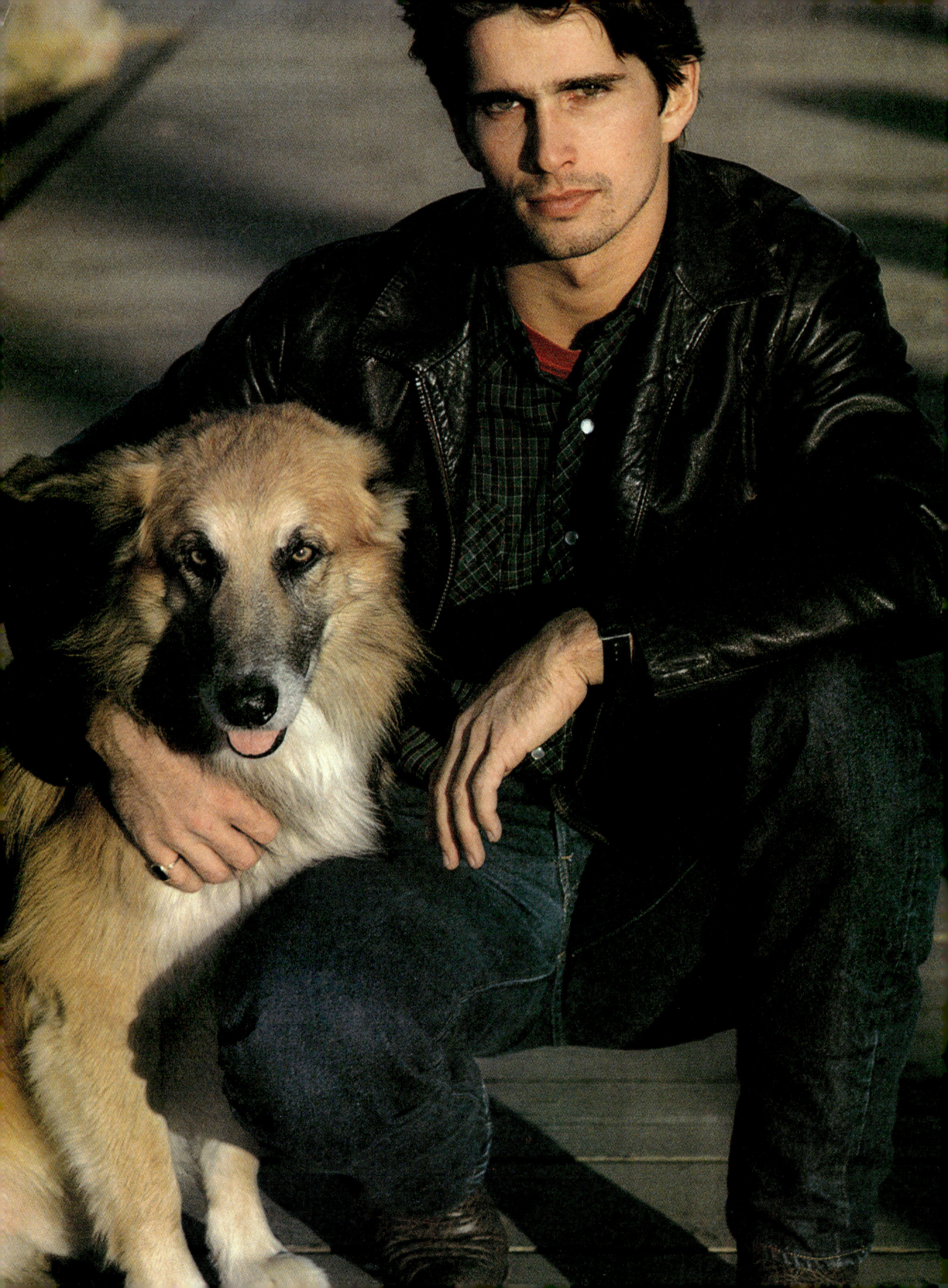

Thom Fleming

Thom Fleming is known as the industry's daredevil. "I have a reputation for doing crazy things," says Thom. "I'm not afraid of much." And certain photo sessions have required Thom to prove his point. He has, for instance, modeled swimsuits at sixty feet under the ocean — without an oxygen tank. For a Tarzan-type setup, he once held a female model over a forty-foot precipice. In his most celebrated act of derring-do, Thom wrestled with an eight-foot alligator during a shoot in the Everglades.

"It wasn't a *tame* alligator, either," recalls Thom. "And it wasn't trained. There's nothing *trained* about those suckers. It was a wild, thrashing, mean, rip-your-leg-off alligator. The photographer suggested I do a photo with the 'gator. I grabbed his tail and his mouth. My neck was straining and the veins were ripping out of my arms. The photographer called out, 'Come on, Thom, *smile*.' He was up on a four-foot platform. It was easy for *him* to smile."

Where does Thom Fleming see himself in the world of high fashion? "I think I'm basically a character," he says. "I'm comic relief. That doesn't mean I'm not serious about getting the shot. But when I get on a job, I like to make it as much fun as I can. That's my job, to make everything easier."

Thom's dark handsomeness has caused him to be labeled "a swarthy type" in the business, but that monicker disturbs Thom. "In pictures," he says, "I come across as a young executive, and I look four or five years younger than I am. But there are very few photographs in which I'm myself. Few photographers capture me — or want to." Those pictures that most closely capture Thom's personality are "casual, relaxed, nothing pretentious, nothing stylized," he says. The picture may have him fishing or romping with a dog or even wrestling with an alligator — "doing something absolutely stupid, which is probably me."

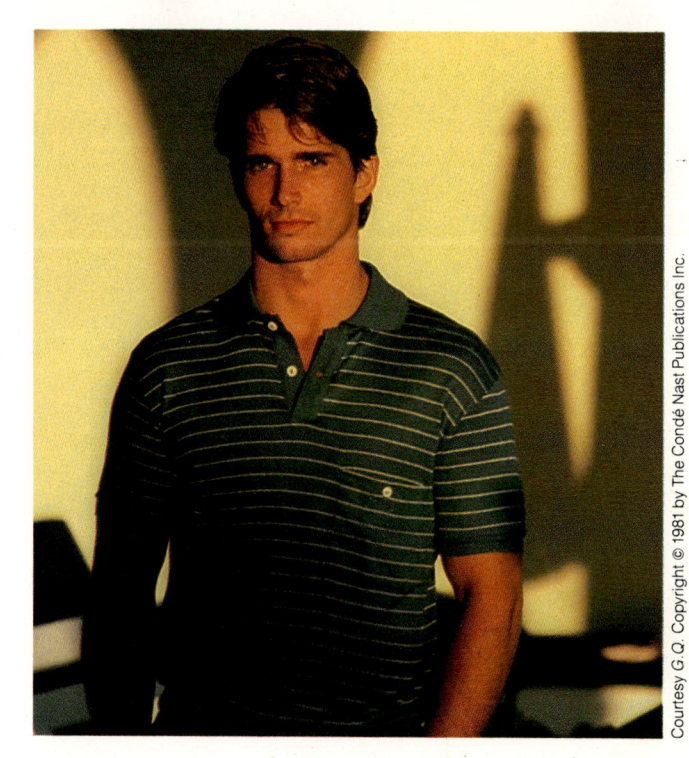

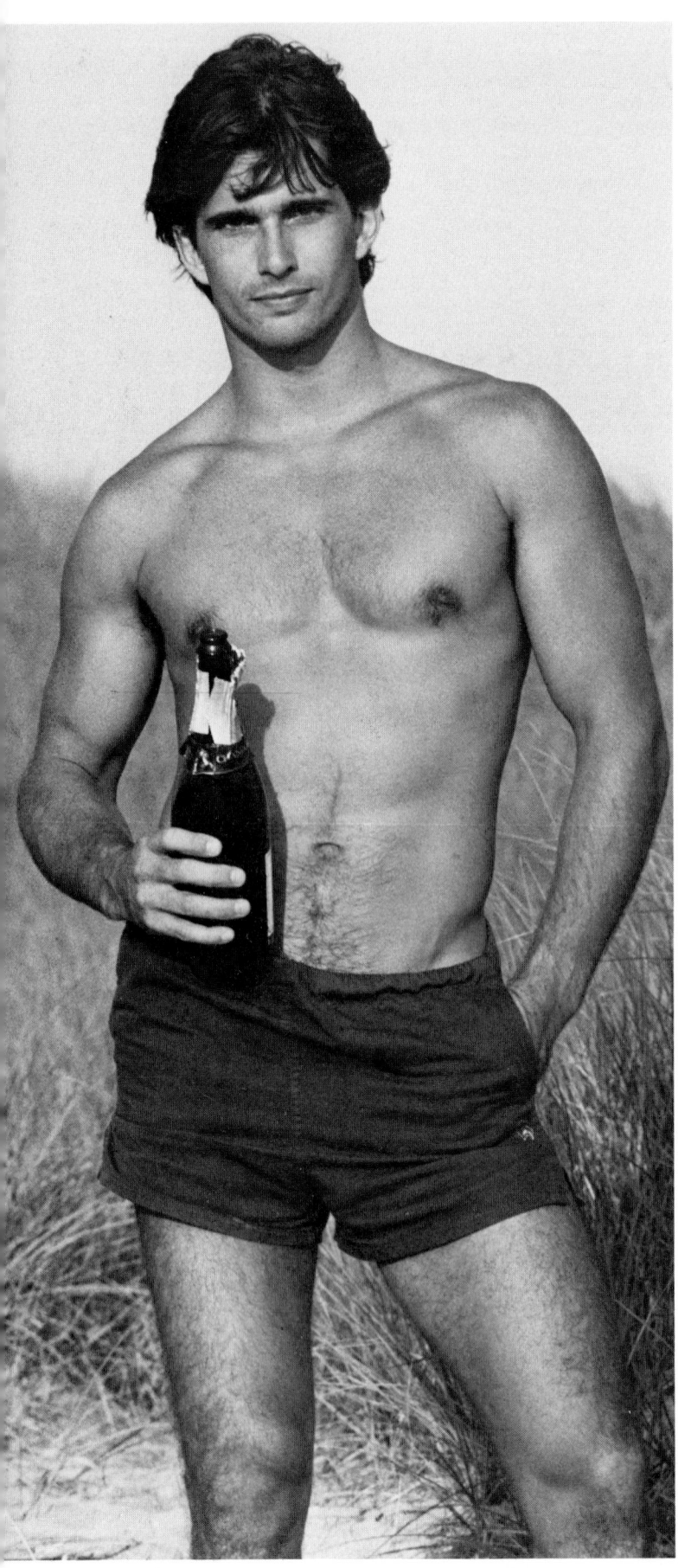

> "When you've lived on potatoes for a month, as I did once, you appreciate what you're doing when you're a model. I make more in a minute now than I did in an hour at my old jobs."

Despite his sardonic, wisecracking streak, there's a serious side to Thom Fleming. Because he didn't begin modeling until he was twenty-eight and widely experienced, Thom has a down-to-earth perspective on his high-profile career. "A lot of people come into this field right out of high school and college," he says. "They never did anything before, and they burn out on being fed, dressed, cared for. All of a sudden, they get out in a world that doesn't treat people that way, and they freak." Thom believes earlier occupations helped him handle his current career more soundly. Thom majored in biology at Wagner College, and has worked as a clammer, a carpenter, and a paramedic — that last profession in particular has influenced his view of the world. "When you've seen a buddy D.O.A. or you've run into a burning house to save somebody, or you've seen a woman giving birth, you have the whole gamut. It gives you a different angle on things. I've dealt with life and death on a real, close, basic level." Even though he now works full-time as a model, Thom has kept his certification as a paramedic "for my own head." Says Thom, "Modeling is *part* of my life, not my whole life. I still get my emotional and mental release working on the ambulance."

Thom's discovery as a model is a genuine Cinderella story. A native of Amityville, New York (on Long Island), Thom was clamming for a caterer in Montauk when an acquaintance suggested that he consider modeling. He halfheartedly pursued the notion, getting some test shots taken. "I did it as a goof," he says. Within six weeks, however, Thom had shot a *GQ* cover, a spread for *Men's Bazaar Italia,* and done work for Valentino and Calvin Klein. "I fell into modeling," observes Thom, "and if it hadn't happened that way, I wouldn't have gone into it. I never felt I was good-looking. I never gave my looks much credence. When I was voted best-looking in high school, I thought it was a bad joke."

When Thom did his first test shots, he was twenty-five pounds heavier than his current weight. He dropped twenty pounds before his first booking, but maintained his solid muscularity. At the time of his first shot, he fit into a size 44 jacket instead of a model's usual 40 regular. Recalls Thom, "They gave me a 40 regular, and when I went to button it, the shirt ripped. It had to be slit to fit me." To keep what he calls "the more average physique" that a model needs to fit the client's clothes, Thom no longer works out — to his great frustration. "I ride my bike everywhere, but boy, do I miss the weights. It took me a long time to get used to my old head in a new body." Thom lives in a fifth-floor-walk-up apartment on Manhattan's East Side, but as often as possible, he retreats to Montauk, Long Island, where he has bought property and plans to build a home.

In addition to modeling, Thom is seriously pursuing a career as an actor. He has signed a development deal with ABC, and he is studying now in New York. "My classic line," he says, "is 'I've been acting for thirty years, why shouldn't I get paid for it?' But in fact, I think I have a lot of experience I could draw on for a character. I'm sensitive and I'm very aware of my feelings, and I think I could do television or movies or even stage." But whatever daredevil thing Thom does next, it will certainly reflect his personal philosophy. "It's very important for me to maintain my integrity in what I do," he says. "What makes a person is not his face but his heart and his head."

Thomas Fleming
Vital & Not So Vital Statistics
Birthdate: August 18, 1952
Height: 6'1"
Weight: 175 lbs.
Hair: Brown
Eyes: Hazel
Personal Favorites —
Actress: Mae West
Actors: Harrison Ford; William Hurt
Vacation Spot: Mustique, in the Caribbean
Snack: Clams (fresh)
Drink: Budweiser beer
Town: Montauk
Hangouts: Montauk Point; and Jim McMullen's, Tokubei, Oren and Aretsky, all in New York City
TV Shows: *Barney Miller; M*A*S*H*
Cartoons: *Popeye; Betty Boop*
Movie: *Fantasia*
Hobbies: Working out on Nautilus; carpentry; softball
Time of Day: Dusk; dawn
Moisturizer and Shaving Cream: Kiehl's
Agency: Ford, New York City

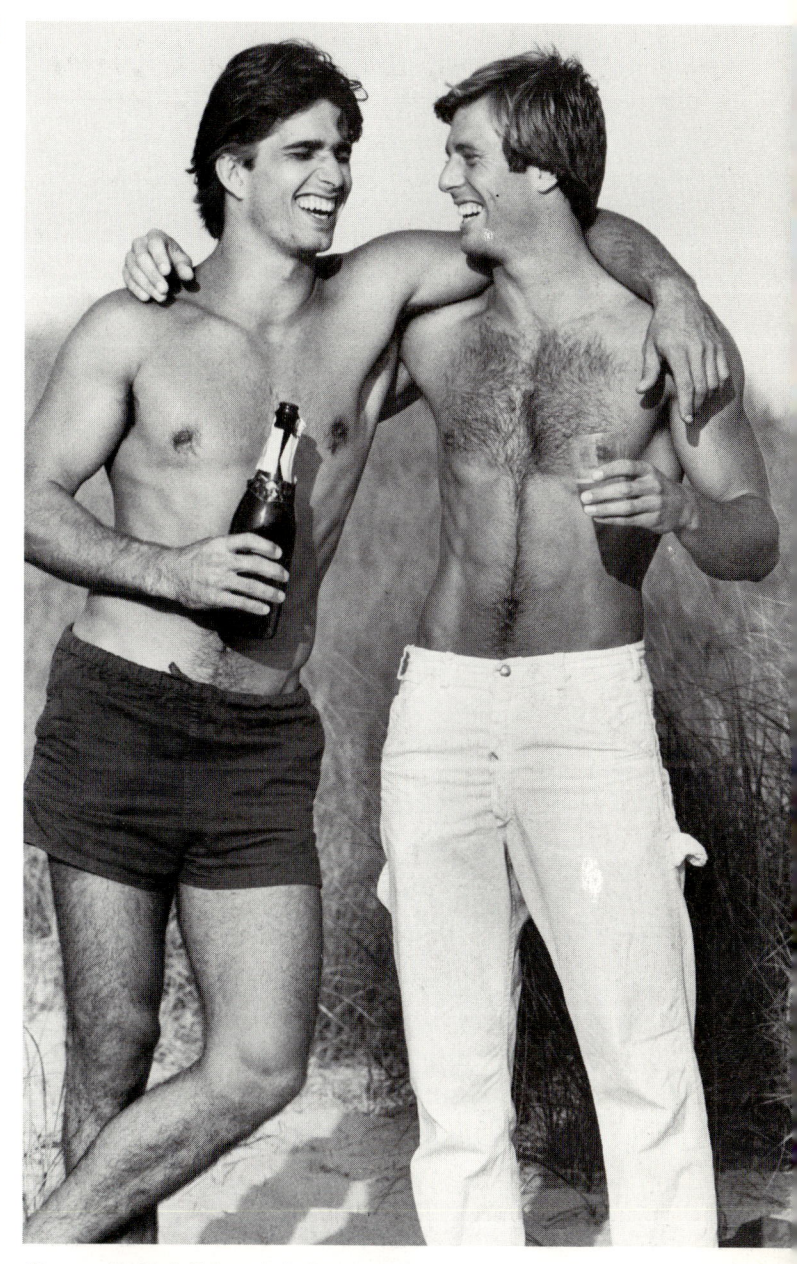

Thom with Rick Edwards in Southampton

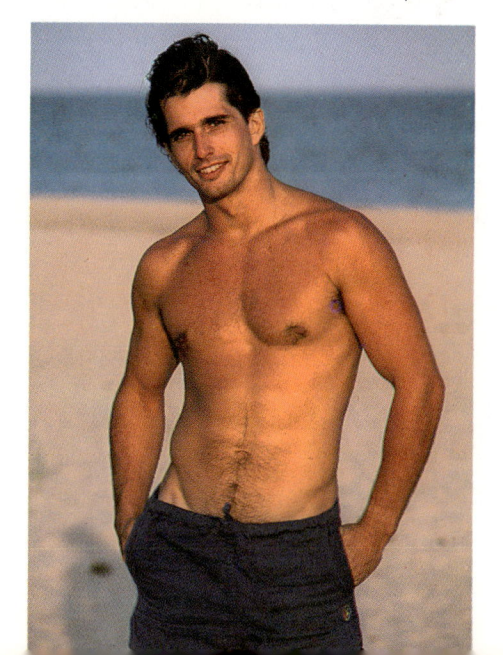

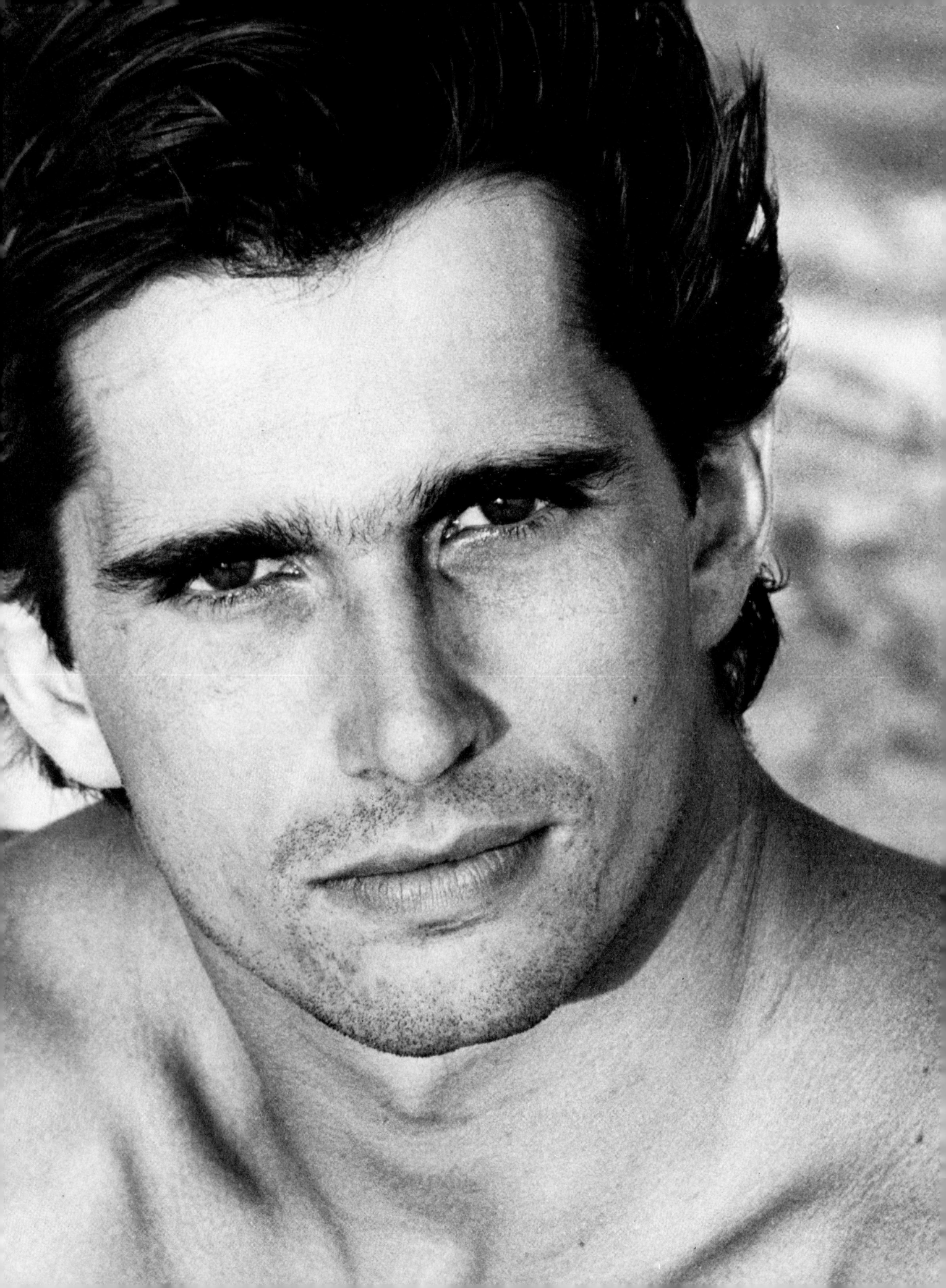

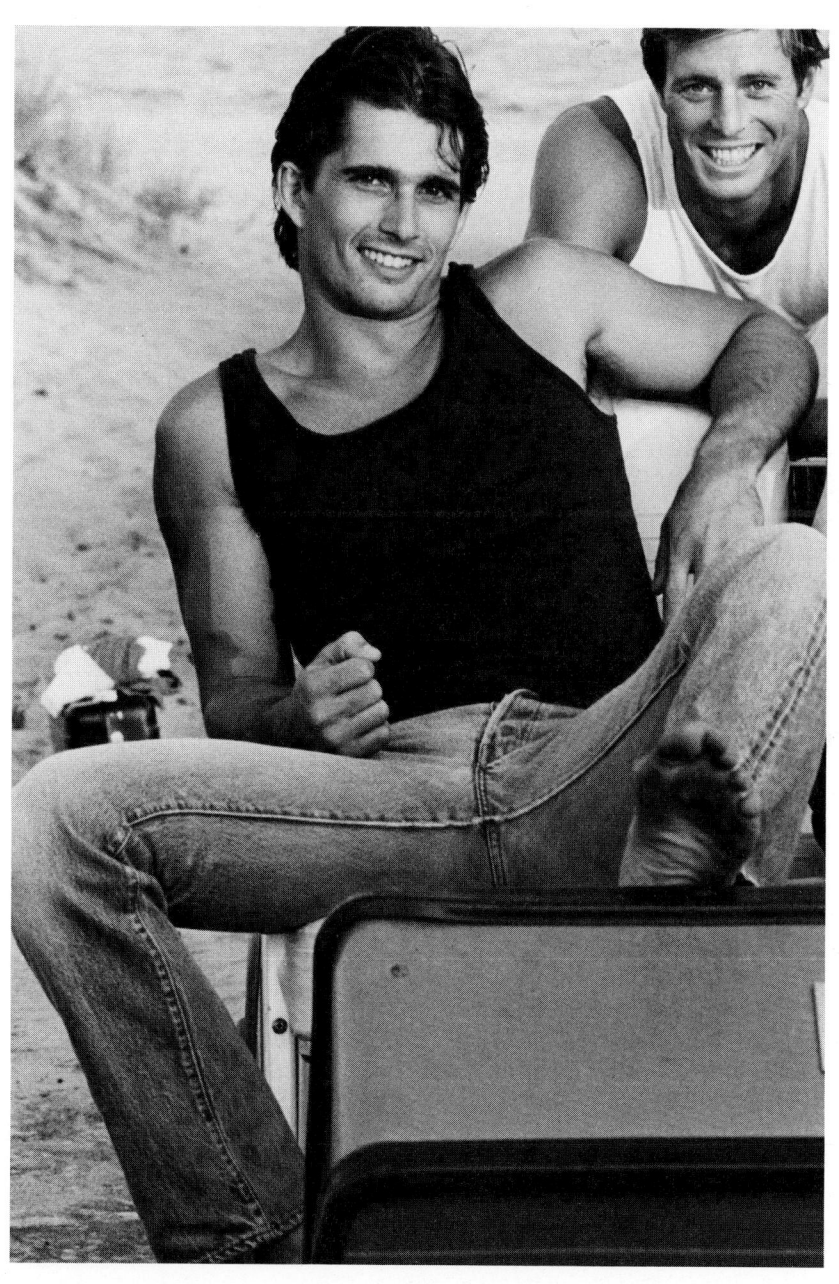

"I definitely want to have your basic 2.2 kids and a white house and a white picket fence somewhere with a lot of land underneath it, hopefully in Montauk. I want to have a family. I'm feeling very paternal lately."

Acknowledgments

Patrick Freydberg's creative input and contribution to the production of this book made the difference. I am indebted to Joe Hunter, Vice President of the Ford Agency, for his continuous encouragement. I am also grateful to: Channa Taub, my editor at NAL, for her support and contribution; Merrilee Heifetz, my agent at Writer's House, whose belief in me was invaluable; Robert Luzzi, my designer, for lending his creative talents to the project; and Josh Reid, whose writing illuminated the individual personalities in each of the profiles. Special thanks to:

Gary Schultz, my photographic assistant
Michael Pantaleoni, Esq.
Charlotte Hardy, my mother
Crystie and Varda Hardy, my sisters
Laurence P. Mitchell
Marco Glaviano
Robert Brown
Jesse Kornbluth
Lorna Koski
Scot Haller
Pauline Elias
Marianne Goodman
Michele Pierson
Guy McCarter
Victoria Wisdom
Vincent Fremont
Nina Blanchard Agency, Los Angeles
Ford Agency, New York
Click Agency, New York
Zoli Agency, New York
Wilhelmina Agency, New York
Eric Forrest
The Kuhns in California, for their unending hospitality
Bruce Weber, whose photographs have served both as an innovation in men's fashion photography and as a personal inspiration